D0122823

Out of Joint

American Lives

Series editor: Tobias Wolff

Out of Joint

A Private & Public
Story of Arthritis

Mary Felstiner

UNIVERSITY OF NEBRASKA PRESS

LINCOLN • LONDON

"Casing My Joints: A Public and Private
Story of Arthritis," reprinted from
Feminist Studies 26, no. 2
(Summer 2000): 273–85.
Used with permission of the publisher,
Feminist Studies, Inc.

The lines from
"Contradictions: Tracking Poems,"
copyright 2002, 1986, by Adrienne Rich,
from *The Fact of a Doorframe:*
Selected Poems 1950–2001
by Adrienne Rich. Used by permission
of the author and
W. W. Norton & Company, Inc.

♾

Library of Congress Cataloging-in-Publication Data
Felstiner, Mary Lowenthal, 1941–
Out of joint : a private and public story
of arthritis / Mary Felstiner.
p. cm.—(American lives)
Includes bibliographical references.
ISBN-13: 978-0-8032-2030-0 (cloth : alk. paper)
ISBN-10: 0-8032-2030-8 (cloth : alk. paper)
1. Felstiner, Mary Lowenthal, 1941—Health.
2. Rheumatoid arthritis—Patients—Biography.
I. Title.   II. Series.
RC933.F45 2005
362.196'7227'0092—dc22
2005008093

Set in Quadraat and Quadraat Sans by Kim Essman.
Designed by R. W. Boeche.
Printed by Maple-Vail.

for John and for Ruth
from the heart

I am poured out like water,
and all my bones are out of joint.
Psalm 22:15

The time is out of joint.
Hamlet 1.5.206

Contents

Illustrations

Acknowledgments

If this were a standard autobiography, it would fill up with family and spill over with friends. But following a life through arthritis shows only a portion of it and doesn't do justice to those most essential to me, especially my in-laws, Susan and Didier Thomas, Celia Lowenthal, Scobie Puchtler, and my comadre, Cathy Short; my nieces and nephew, Lia Lowenthal, Katherine Denham, and Daniel Thomas; our aunt Ruth Bendor and the Bendor family; and my friends of the heart, Emily Abel, Guiguite and Joe Frank, Estelle Freedman, Margo Horn, Marion Hunt, Penny Janeway, Toni Kestenbaum, Si Lazarus, Toni Lester, Mary Newmann, Ruth Rosen, Mary Rothschild, Adele Simmons, Nina Jo Smith, Myra Strober, Joan Weimer, Marilyn and Irv Yalom. For their encouragement and affection I feel the deepest gratitude.

Full credit goes to the Nits, a writers' group that started me off and kept me at it: Whitney Chadwick, Carol Field, Diana Ketcham, Diana O'Hehir, Cyra McFadden, Jean McMann, Carol Monpere, BK Moran, Annegret Ogden, and Alison Owings. Among those, Alison, Carol, Carol, Diana O., and Whitney committed brave acts of editing. To my other primary readers, the ones digging deeply into the manuscript, giving generous and thought-provoking help—Emily Abel, Elizabeth Benedict, Alek Felstiner, Sarah Felstiner, Adam Hochschild, Penny Janeway, Gerda Lerner, Olga Seham, Melanie Thernstrom—I offer all my appreciation, and it will never be half enough. Ruth Rosen, Joan Weimer, and John Felstiner deserve lifelong thanks for their splendid editing and loving-kindness, as well as major tax deductions for the many days they took from their own work to see this project through.

Every body and spirit ought to have the outstanding physicians I've relied on, Melvin Britton and Nan Link; the generous assistance of Shana Bernstein, Alison Field, and Camille George; and the fine services of the Office of Disability Programs at San Francisco State University.

With great respect I thank the writers' residencies that supported this project: the Corporation of Yaddo, the Djerassi Foundation, the MacDowell Colony, the Millay Colony, the Hedgebrook Foundation, the Mesa Refuge, and the Institute for Research on Women and Gender at Stanford University. Versions of chapters written at these residencies appeared earlier in *Feminist Studies* (2000); *Inside the American Couple*, edited by Marilyn Yalom and Laura Carstensen (2002); and *The Politics of Women's Bodies: Sexuality, Appearance, and Behavior*, edited by Rose Weitz (2002).

I'm indebted as well to a remarkable agent, Gail Hochman; an outstanding editor, Ladette Randolph; an astute copyeditor, Carol Sickman-Garner; and a spirited, on-the-ball staff at the University of Nebraska Press.

Though the events recounted are true, drawn from private letters, diaries, and medical files, as well as research libraries, I did take a few liberties, braiding discussions together, omitting or altering names or features for privacy. I treat memoir as a form of history, but conversations are approximations, and no amount of effort, at times, can make memory strictly reliable.

Because a personal story involves those who are closest, my deepest recognition goes to Sarah, Alek, and John Felstiner, the ones I'm forever grateful to be joined with.

I begin, in the morning, by casing my joints. I spot-check my ankles on the stairs, flex my fingers at the kitchen counter, hope to peel an orange or open a jar, give up trying. Too stiff today.

These same joints used to glide through my rooms from morning to midnight, tossing off letters or scooping out chocolate ripple. I was still young, in my twenties, at the time they suddenly turned old. Then from one day to the next my life got thrown out of joint. An ailment called rheumatoid arthritis took hold of me, along with two million other people, mostly women. It felt like fire and ice, making my joints flare and congeal. It pinioned the moving parts and wrecked the bones' soft cushions. It demanded tablets and shots, baths to soak in, helpers to lean on, until no other remedy—please, no suggestions—seemed worth trying. My goal was to last it out, nothing more.

Of the countless people bearing daylong, lifelong ailments, a surprising portion live with a hundred kinds of arthritis. Some of them hardly move till midday, their pain's that bad. Others gulp down pills and take the side effects. Some have surgeons scrape their bones or replace joints. Others quit their jobs or bring home a fraction of what they'd earn if their joints worked right. Some feel jolted out of time, young but old. Others watch their lives coming apart at any age. Some whine and moan. Others are struck dumb. Most go without saying much about it. And at one time or another all these people were me.

For thirty years I kept my life-with-arthritis under wraps. The reason, I'm ashamed to say, was shame. I was embarrassed to ask for favors on the job, chagrined at moving slower than full stride, humbled by looking tired and antique. What's worse, I judged my slowness as a fault, marking myself tardy every day, behind the curve.

Before this disease I'd always sped forward, pushed by desire, will, and pride (I never thought of joints) through college and halfway through grad school, heading toward history teaching, raising a baby too. I'd jumped into the women's movement and helped create a feminist icon—the invincible, independent woman—that I couldn't imitate after arthritis set in. I still held to my former desires and aims, just chewed myself out for falling short of them.

Waking with arthritis and going to sleep with it, for decades, I learned to shrink before that icon. Even now, with great drugs, I'm tired, pained, slower than anyone realizes. Producing a meal, a memo, let alone an actual paragraph, means measuring out every move. I'm OK to hike, but short on velocity or traction. Fine to make sandwiches, but bad with grip, with twist tops. Good for an hour of gabbing, but hopeless with handwriting or typing.

During the early years I tried pretty hard to learn nothing about my disease, certainly not why it came to me in the first place. Grasping at causes seemed so fruitless I hit on only one insight: it wasn't going to go away. In fact I barely said the name *rheumatoid arthritis* out loud.

For others too the varied experience of arthritis—stiffening, harrowing, immense—remains privately told or more likely untold. Oddly absent from public space is any sustained personal story (one I needed but never could find). This story belongs to millions of Americans with connective-tissue diseases like rheumatoid arthritis, osteoarthritis, fibromyalgia, some of them pesky and persistent, some exceedingly painful, some more treatable than many think, some more shameful than they should be, all unpublicized at best by those who live inside them. Now that arthritis drugs get pushed onto and whipped off the market, more publicly than ever before, we know enough to ask (for the first time in history) how bad arthritis is and what should be done, at what cost, for its sufferers. But no answers will come unless we have someone's full personal disclosure about the disease.

If arthritis sufferers still find it tough to confess, that's because their condition has stayed obscured from view. For most of my years few news stories covered the extent of arthritis, few fresh drugs alleviated its pains, few new doctors specialized in treating it. Meanwhile long inattention made the condition worse than it needed to be.

Few people, even now, realize that one in three Americans have arthritis, upward of seventy million adults (most with osteoarthritis, a disease wearing down cartilage between bones), plus three hundred thousand children. Arthritis isn't known for what it is, our nation's most common disease, more hurtful and impairing, more costly (eighty-two billion dollars in annual impact), more rampant than anyone admits.

I'm forced to ask: how has it become possible to treat a national curse like a private mishap and a personal shame?

If I want this question on the table along with everything else, I have to change my mind about joints. By medical lights mine present a case of common degeneration. Even drugs that work are basically flame retardants, slowing damage but never stopping it. In chronic terms I have nothing to look forward to but a steady downward spiral. Yet slowly I'm arriving at another view, a view that harm is done, over time, by leaving illnesses unspoken and that good might come of knowing the ingenuity it takes to deal with them.

The upshot is, I'm trying to heal by delving into history. Not that visiting the past erases the pain of having lived there: it doesn't equal cure and isn't promoted by the AMA. Yet tracing a private timeline, and splicing it into a public one, has been the single best discovery of my chronic years, a way of enduring that's more like a way of moving ahead.

With a long illness there's time to do the thing historians do: sleuth around, go back to the sources, dig up old diaries stashed in the attic, recall the years before the disease hit, scan medical files kept under lock and key, pick through pieces of the past, reclaim a body that could have been ditched. Anyone can do it—pry open medical secrets, forgotten life events, and memories that witness the times. It's never too late to lift the limbs an inch or two by breathing the past back into them.

In the afternoon I swear, "I can take this, damn it," punching a two-hundred-dollar syringe, a wonder drug, into my thigh. I can take this weekly shot, the sequel of all-over hives, the future side effects—anything to push back the pain. Anything to climb the hills behind my house so a light wind can brush my skin.

Climbing today I can see the liberty I'm all for, and up against, as joggers and striders, sports bras and stretch pants, speed past me and my somewhat hidden handicap. Of course *handicap* isn't the proper word anymore: it sounds accusing, like faulting people themselves instead of the barriers that get in their way. But it also sounds refreshing, seeming to level unearned advantages, offer slower people a head start, faster ones a little responsibility. For years I've been imagining an arbiter called the Angel of Anatomy, who'll balance everyone's chances, worsen an ailment here or grant a remission there. I've even made a bizarre bargain with this Angel: in exchange for hushed-up arthritis on my part, nothing dreadful can happen to my family.

Recently I've been granted a breather, released from stiffness by way of drugs. This remission arrived like new grass over last year's straw, a temporary state (who knows what's next?) where people like me hope to live out a lifetime. After years of dragging up these paths, now my joints are pretty much striding along. And I'm stunned by how much effort—medical and social, as well as personal—it's taken to get them moving.

Now's a good time to recall which efforts, over the years, managed to get my joints through the trials of being a parent, a teacher, a writer, a walker. From the start I relied on the empathy of family and friends. Then I tried research, learning where arthritis attacks the body, what causes inflammation, stiffness, fatigue, and danger. Eventually I got more daring, plunging into self-help and feminism, struggling with technology and alternative treatments, risking new remedies. Finally I've come far enough to track this long transformation.

Under an old familiar oak, an Endurance Tree, straining for straightness as if an unseen water table feeds its branches, I look on my bent joints with new curiosity. Which treatments and attitudes fed into them? Which beliefs kept blaming sickness on inborn defects or self-made faults? Why did silence take hold of this illness, and why is it beginning to expire? What changed recently so that "The Coming Epidemic of Arthritis" now rates cover stories in *Time* and *Newsweek*? What is forcing my ailment, and myself with it, into the open? What leaps in technology, what drives for remedies or profits, and above all what movements for rights have started to turn my shame upside down?

Only by incorporating all these changes—how much it took to get me to this place on this day—can the ankles and knees and toes and shoulders and elbows and hips and hands and neck and back and wrists and knuckles make their way toward healing.

Healing by history calls for an experiment. It has to do with binding to-gether the pieces I've picked from my past, the same way joints connect the bones. If I think of others whose bodies keep backsliding, if my own questions can help them view illness in fresh ways, then I'll keep asking about my past: what did it set me up for? And about prospects: what happened to everything I expected? What changed my lot—new drugs, new rights? What about family? Did it prop me up, or did I drag it down? And pain: how much could I take? And the choices I made: any lucky ones? And despair: could I draw any good out of it?

In this experiment I hope to link my own moving parts with motions in public life and become, after years of silence, someone who speaks up about bodies in trouble, who changes the way trouble is privatized. Because my joints can't do what they used to, they might get me going this new way.

As evening sun lights the hilltop, I come on a flock of blackbirds roost-ing. A moment later, startled by wind, they burst into breakaway flight, and I feel lifted among them. I turn and head across a ridge, the wind catching me too, pasting my T-shirt around my ribs, moving my heavy feet along. I'm about to take a flyer, about to take a chance on the worst that's happened making the best sense of my life.

To lay open that life, I could begin anywhere, from my birth in a health-filled family to the deaths of all but me. But a juncture at midpoint is where I'll start off, thinking back to one late-night moment, in 1969.

There I am, in my twenties and sound asleep, when a first warning of pain like a sudden storm comes rolling in on me.

Out of Joint

I. Getting Hurt

I feel signified by pain.

Adrienne Rich,
The Fact of a Doorframe

Shock, 1969

Hours before morning I wake feeling my wrists starched. What is this? And scorched. What is this?

A dawn wind slaps the shutter against a stucco wall. A Southern Pacific train keens at a crossing. Our baby startles and whimpers. A rasp comes from somewhere, probably from me.

The next minute John leans over me, thin as a splinter, asking, "You OK, love?"

"*Damn* it, would you stop that hammering?"

"It's just the shutter."

"It's my wrists. Someone's hammering them."

"What?"

"I don't know what."

Tiny Sarah, light of my life, squirms to be fed, but her small bones weigh like ingots on my lower arms. I must have strained my wrists lifting her a good eight hours a day to nurse. I lift again, as if love's effortless, like fear. I breathe her scalp. John breathes mine.

Soon morning sun fools with the thermostat and pulls wind off San Francisco Bay into our rooms. By then it's time for me to LEAVE, I shout, for WORK, as I've been raised to call what goes on in a library. I don't have leisure today for . . . whatever this hammering is. Today has to get me a few pages nearer to the end of a graduate thesis so I can step into some college as a licensed history teacher. No interruptions except from the light of my life, and this morning she'll shine in a babysitter's house.

I need something quick, like Ace bandages or maybe wrist splints. But in the examining room at the Palo Alto Clinic an on-call doctor studies my arms and says something odd. He's sending me for blood tests.

Just splint the wrists, OK?

"Let's help them heal," he says and shoots them up with Novocain, then cortisone.

I already know they won't heal if I'm holding an infant all the time.

"John?" I call as soon as he's home from teaching comic literature at Stanford, balancing Sarah plus diaper bag on his forearms. "Where's that feeding schedule we made last week?" John finds it and reads: "2:10, 5:15, 7:30, 11:45, 3:30, 6:30, 9:30, 12:30. Colic: 6:30, 9:30, midnight, 4:15, 7:45." No wonder my wrists take a beating.

So I consider things to cut out. The history thesis I keep flailing at? The dinnertime and cleanup with John? The nursing and lifting and rocking I'd rather do or die? After two weeks of all this, plus pain, I'm referred to a specialist, a Dr. B., whose framed diploma boldfaces a word I don't like the look of.

Rheumatology.

And here's a knock, his head around the door, a nod at my slender chart. "So, you do graduate work on Latin America?" And then, "Your lab results are in." Pause. "Your rheumatoid factor is positive." Pause. "Your sedimentation rate is elevated—"

"That sounds up and running."

But I see in his face I've come down with something bad.

"Most likely," he says, "it's rheumatoid arthritis," a name that's all new to me. I shiver in my flimsy clinic gown and watch Dr. B.'s sharp eyes for clues. What he offers next is lucid, though too strange to reach my brain: " . . . joints stiffen . . . inflamed membranes thicken . . . erode cartilage . . ." Then he shakes a new ballpoint like a thermometer, tears off the first page of a prescription pad, and writes "PTX6." The ballpoint clicks shut. Not many prescriptions come my way, yet this one decodes easily: Physical Therapy Six Times. Nothing I can't handle.

But the instant my palm turns over to take the prescription, a sharpness bites my wrist. After lifting, grasping, reaching, seizing for twenty-eight years, the person under my skin discovers she uses joints. My privilege was making a move and never caring how. To think this can be taken away by inflamed little membranes, thick as thieves.

I'm ready to leave on the spot, but he's ready to talk. "Aspirin," he says, "will be our ally."

Our? He's joining me?

"We'll use astronomic doses against inflammation."

I shrug. Aspirin. Big deal.

"Later we might move up to stronger drugs."

We again, and *later*: he's offering a long-term contract. My head shakes. No drugs for me, no later.

He waits a minute, then nods briskly. "Any questions?"

I stay still, sure that this body should be caring for a baby and not its own bones. His hand reaches to shake mine and lays a brochure there. I glance at it, then sit down in the waiting room. The first thing I learn is that "arthritis" is a disease between bone and bone. With sudden nausea I visualize a skeleton inside me, motionless as death, only lifted and moved by my joints: so joints are life itself. Then I learn arthritis stands for more than one hundred different diseases. It comes from *arth*, joint, plus *itis*, inflammation. Just seeing these italics, I have to lay emphasis on kinder words. "Arthritis *sometimes* causes stiffness, pain and swelling. In some people, only a *few* joints are affected and the impact may be *small*. In others, the entire body *may* be affected. Arthritis may be chronic, which means it *could* last on and *off* for as long as a lifetime."

"Stiffness" scares me. So does "swelling" and worst of all "pain." I keep rereading these words, but the ones poised to spring later don't even reach my mind. *Chronic*, the paragraph slips in at the end. *Lifetime*.

It takes me a full week with that brochure to realize it's an eviction notice. Give up what was your body. And don't ask for it back.

The next day, in a hand-me-down armchair, I pull the baby close, stare out at a willow bending easy limbs, and make an awful guess: that the best and worst events—new baby, new blood test—have some reason for happening at the same time. I don't ask what the reason is.

Settling Sarah in her carrier, I turn to a wedding gift from three years ago, the dependable *Britannica*. At "Arthritis" I stop acting like a grown-up and sprawl on the rug, the way I nosed into the *World Book* for fifth-grade reports. Back then I was growing up in an industrial city that looked to my eyes more like a village of medicine men. In Pittsburgh lived Dr. Salk and Dr. Spock, village friends of my family, so I expected

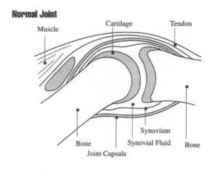

Normal Joint

Muscle — Cartilage — Tendon

Synovium
Bone — Synovial Fluid — Bone
Joint Capsule

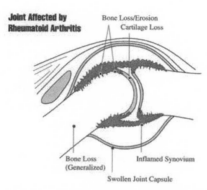

Joint Affected by Rheumatoid Arthritis

Bone Loss/Erosion
Cartilage Loss

Bone Loss (Generalized) — Inflamed Synovium
Swollen Joint Capsule

Illustration courtesy of the National Institute of Arthritis and Musculoskeletal and Skin Diseases Information Clearinghouse.

no trouble with my body. It would simply grow and prosper and be married to.

I assumed well-being, or at least the smoothing of ills, until this moment. Now my mind gets busy and talks to itself about new realities:

How long does this last?

A lifetime.

It won't go away?

It's incurable.

I'll just get worse?

And worse.

Will I get crippled?

And then some.

Meaning—?

Pain.

But it's not life-threatening.

Umm . . .

It is?

I grab the phone, knowing the moment has come to interrupt John in his Stanford office, where students are asking him to explain comic absurdity.

"Oh, hi," he says. "Where are you?"

"Uh, home?" For full effect I pull the phone to where the baby's starting to cry. "I'm reading awful stuff on arthritis. How could I get this disease? I'm young. I haven't done anything bad yet. And now my feet burn."

"Oh no. No."

"It's slipping downward, I think."

"I'll be there."

"I *am* there."

Nuzzling the baby's neck, I count six joints of mine—wrists, elbows, shoulders, the joints for toting a baby—now fritzed by a fast-moving disease. I count again because I love this job. I want to keep it. But if being a mother isn't jollying a baby, isn't scooping a toddler from the stairs and fetching each toy heaved from the highchair, isn't tumbling and racing a preschooler, and so on from there, then what's left?

I lever the baby and an Evenflo bottle into the crib, twisting my wrists. What's left is my own mother's way of raising me all studious, which led down the line to the thesis I'm so anxious about. No, I want to become a rough-and-tumble playtime parent, the kind John gets to be.

Minutes later, as he bounds up the stairs to take over, I recall us just months ago, newly minted parents, leaning on each other, delighted to divide any labor (after birth labor) half and half. Our motto was *fair's fair*. Now our contract has one little add-on we never signed. A disease is butting in. Forget fifty-fifty. I don't know how we're going to make it work when fair isn't fair anymore.

Six months into illness I don't even see how I'm going to finish grad school. Heading to the Stanford library one day, I wonder if I look like a person in distress. Of course I do. I'm a joint disorder making its way across a parking lot. Tugging the library doors, first with one hand, then both, I silently answer anyone curious as to what the trouble is. First imagine a well-made gear between two bones. A handy capsule surrounds it, holds it steady. Spongy cartilage makes it flexible and smooth. High-grade fluid lubricates it. Fibrous ligaments keep its motion sensible, so knees don't twirl or fingers skitter. Now imagine a multiform disease messing with any of this. It would ruin the whole moving part.

I almost wish I had the most common form of the disease, osteoarthritis, which seems as natural as aging: over time cartilage breaks down between bones. Osteoarthritis chips at knees or spine or hips or fingers, letting bones grate against each other, loosen particles, lock and hurt. All this happens in my kind of arthritis too, but with different joints: wrists and elbows and shoulders, my instruments for writing and for raising a child. In my rheumatoid kind look how both arms stiffen, and both legs. See the symmetry. Osteoarthritis goes for a hand here, a hip there, degenerative and choosy. Rheumatoid fastens on anything that flexes. Most people struggling with heavy doors have osteoarthritis, but in this country over two million have my kind, fifty million worldwide, and I don't know even one of them—well, one. Rheumatoid is the second most common and the worst form of arthritis (I've read this in a clinic brochure), a systemic chronic disabling incurable painful wasting disease. Also autoimmune. It keeps treating body parts as aliens, keeps rousing immune cells until they're attacking familiars as suspects, picking on bones they're supposed to be keeping safe.

Pulling out a heavy library chair, my wrists pop, along with a premise—that joints are born for quiet service, like Jeeves. Why did mine turn against me at just this point? The question latches onto one I'm following today for my thesis, on Chile at Independence. Why did the "joints" of a body politic rebel—the magistrates whose "sickness" was "sedition" (in Thomas Hobbes's words)? To my eyes Hobbes's terms expose a system warping under pressure. Defective joints defect.

Defective joints ruin any self-portrait I have in mind. They give this twenty-something woman a stunned and glazed look. Caption: How will she raise a baby with this damaged body or take up any work again?

Some of the clinic doctors I've seen for their expertise don't quite see mine. Their notes refer to me as a "28 year old professor's wife," a "charming lady," and a "housewife" with RA, as they call rheumatoid arthritis. My own physician seems to see deeper. He's always alert and inquiring, sometimes inviting me into his office when he dictates my medical chart: "She has been very tense and under a great deal of distress as a result of this diagnosis. She thinks this has made her arthritis worse and I would certainly be prepared to agree."

I ask him, "Is the tension that obvious?" He says yes, lightly squeezing right and left elbows. "And you're tired. Fatigue goes along with RA." I turn away: it's too much for me, his naming symptoms I can't afford.

"Should I . . ." But I'm about to ask if I should have prevented this somehow. "Should I do something more?"

"Keep taking that aspirin. And see the physical therapist."

"I've been putting it off."

A week later a rehab room in Stanford Hospital welcomes me with fluorescent tubes flickering over steam-gray linoleum and orange plastic seats. A sweat-suited middle-aged man stands on a mat and ratchets side to side, whining softly at each arc. In his joints' robotic clicking I hear, with dismay, my body-to-be. Then unexpectedly he grins. "Takes me all day to loosen up!" he says. Jesus, that's loose?

Abruptly a physical therapist orders, "Dip," and lowers my wrist into a foot-long tub of hot paraffin. When the shimmering tallow forms a thick wax glove, its heat stuns my fingers, and the joints drop in temperature, trying to cool the skin. "Keep dipping."

"For how long?"

"About fifteen minutes."

"In my life, I mean."

"From now on."

"No one's ever done with arthritis?"

Man in sweat suit: "Arthritis? You're so young."

"Yeah, rheumatoid arthritis starts young. It's all topsy-turvy." I'm thinking: up to now, attacca was my move, the way musicians press on without a break, the way I started Stanford grad school straight out of Harvard and Columbia, the way I pumped through a Pittsburgh high school after a progressive elementary and a rough urban primary, and before that nursery school, where I crammed snack. Last year I was stepping toward a new life with a baby, a final degree. Now the moving parts act sluggish, sealed in wax.

As I dip both hands again, I'm begging silently, Turn it back the way it was. Back two years, when I trusted these hands to lift eighteenth-century tomes in Chilean archives, grab onto poles in Santiago's careening buses, grasp partners in Rio's Carnival, grip deck rails on an Amazon steamer, hold John at night in six South American republics. The loss of handiness makes me so sorrowful and mad I peel off the paraffin, wave my heat-flexed fingers at Madame Tussaud here, and rush home.

There I find Sarah whimpering toward a nap. Happily I stroke her back a thousand times until she's asleep and then turn to John. He's grading papers at our shared plywood desk when I fold my arms over him.

"Oh my." He's on his feet. "What's this? More physical therapy?" His fingers run down my spine.

"I just saw the future. It has wax gloves." I pull out his T-shirt and reach up his long back, swivel at his shoulder, and that's when my wrist snaps. One snap tells me this easy impulse won't ever be easy again.

It occurs to me, because it has to, that I'm going to get tight-lipped about RA. I'm gearing up for a job search and can't have anyone knowing what my rheumatologist knows: "There has been a gradual decline in her ability to move around and her ability to be active. She has noted the right shoulder has been painful because she has been carrying her child on her right hip. The right elbow has recently become somewhat painful also."

I rely on that right elbow for writing. If it keeps acting up, call off the job search. For the first time since diagnosis I stop to ask: Why this joint? Why one of mine? In the rheumatology waiting room I dig through my purse for paper, extract a grocery receipt, and scribble something so private I never thought it before. It's an offering, an ode:

> Stay with me
> elbow
> don't be scared

off my body
for my baby
came this way
a blessing
too lucky to last
without a bribe.
Elbow
stick it out

I swiftly bury the receipt in a folder because a woman my age lowers
herself into the next seat with two canes, making me not so bad off. If
I could go backward a year, there'd be no sickness at all. But then no
Sarah either. As if I'd give up anything that has her presence in it.

Just then John comes to fetch me home, with Sarah fastened to his
back on a carrier. From an inner door the doctor starts toward my chair.
Like figures in a fable we gather for a moment: Dr. B. who's trying to
rid me of a disease, John (my pacer) who's pulling ahead, Sarah who
deserves a sprightly mother in return for giving joy. And Mary, who
can't imagine where the plot goes next, whether it sees a marriage
through, or a baby's first year, or anything after that.

At this moment a gust blows in from the terrace and brushes the
circle of characters—patient, partner, daughter, doctor. A wind, I'm
absurdly forced to think, of change.

It takes my mind back to the time before the change, to the years
before arthritis and the things they were supposed to lead to.

Tops, 1959–69

The ten years before arthritis were supposed to lead up and up. From the moment I arrived at college I was told: you're tops, one female admitted to classes at Harvard for every three men. But in fact this was the sixties before the "Sixties," and male classmates lived far away, in spacious suites, while Radcliffe girls crowded into separate dorms. There we waited tables and answered phones for free, services beneath our male-born peers. We scuttled past their men-only library, barred from any place where our physiques would disrupt their studying. Even when our minds were invited to the table, our bodies were placed below the salt. We crossed none of their doorsteps except during so-called parietal hours, a few per day, which the college suspended if their grades dropped. We were their punishment. We were their reward. And I approved of this.

Early on in my freshman seminar a guest speaker advised us, "You can't think hard with a hard-on," and I laughed with the boys—how cool! I never thought to question where I fitted into this scheme or whether my "inner space"—as another guest speaker, Erik Erickson, viewed the female psyche—smelled awful and made me dumb. But Erikson did open a momentous idea for me: "March 9, 1960. Psychiatrist Erik Erikson speaks of freedom being the opportunity provided by limits. Even a 'chronic disease,' he tells us, can be used to strengthen positive beliefs." I took that down.

Certain "limits" (but not female ones) I learned to object to. During freshman summer I got a job with the United Steelworkers Union in Pittsburgh, where the rank and file danced with me in bars, then gave me pathology courses about "dirty mines, lousy mills, creeping automation, damned pinkerton, scab fink spies," and worst of all bleeding, coughing, peeling, lifetime illnesses. I couldn't leave all that alone.

I took it into my head to become a medical researcher or maybe a doctor, though I didn't know any women with jobs like that. Since I did know Jonas Salk's Pittsburgh lab, I signed up for weekly lab work at Massachusetts General Hospital. There Dr. Marion Ropes, Medical Woman of the Year, ran something called *rheumatology*, but I was sent to a pathology lab in the basement. "October 24, 1961. I sealed polyethylene bags full of old organs," thousands of extracted organs: how could so many pieces go wrong? One day, auditing an autopsy, I watched a brain delicately pulled from a healthy person, dead at my age, and decided: medical research, definitely.

Except I was a girl. As a girl I desired love, which had to mean I didn't want labs. In my journal: "Harvard is asking me to live a man's life, that is to *do* something with my education. Dr. Salk asked me what were my fondest dreams about myself. I don't have any—well, maybe a white coat? My only real hope is love and marriage."

When he visited Cambridge again, I wrote, "Saw Dr. Salk for a while today, we talked about finding what's right for yourself, and lots of important things." The important things—biology and medicine—held me breathless, but the assignments proved me worst in show. One day I dropped my test tube, weighed the solution along with bits of glass, and actually got correct results, just that once. This fraud drove me to an appointment with the lab director. I had a crucial question to ask.

"I want to work for . . . medicine, for cures. Is there a way without doing labs? I mean, is there any way?" He was brilliant and kindly, and his smile gave hope. My major, maybe my future, hung on his answer. "No," he said.

Simple as that. I signed up for history.

By senior year, in '63, I was stymied as to what to make of myself, so I retreated each day to play a Harvard harpsichord, which my roommate Zaza said I'd marry for being well tempered with good legs. Then one day my private question—whether to get smart (for what job?) or lovely (for what harpsichord?)—was publicly aired by LIFE magazine. It insisted each Radcliffe girl used to be "fine for a debate, maybe, but not for a date," but now was "a real looker, beautiful as well as brainy." In one full-page photo a spotlighted coed seemed to say something dizzy-

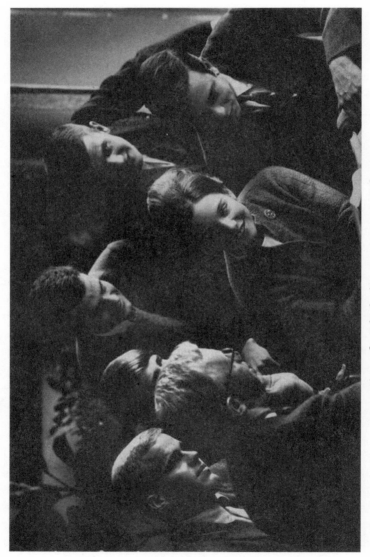

LIFE magazine, 1963; Ted Polumbaum / LIFE magazine / The Newseum.

ing in a seminar of men—actually it showed my favorite professor, my friends, and myself with wide eyes and puffed-up hair. That magazine photo, I was told, advanced my status to a "looker," which made me certain I wasn't anything of the kind. Soon letters began to arrive from panting male readers, until I got a glimmer that "beautiful as well as brainy" wasn't so much a senior-year triumph as a slur.

I felt one-down in each classroom, with its sprinkle of women, thinking all the male students knew their future paths. But I didn't have one—where could girls go?—and might not get chosen to share theirs. I was also beginning to form a notion that reached its full strength six years afterward, with RA. Given "brains and beauty" (as LIFE put it) and a privileged education, I was selfish to mind physical drawbacks like my gender or later my joints. Meanwhile the strain of not minding made me so unsure of myself that my parents had to write, "Junior Phi Beta Kappa didn't come to you unearned." I wrote back admitting to "bitten fingernails and ten extra pounds and crying in Widener stacks and desperate escapism." Even when my adviser sent a note saying, "It's a known fact that you're beautiful, you're smart, so you really shouldn't be anxious!" I scribbled on the back, "I think I'm going to crack."

In that last year of college I clipped articles about depression but filed them separately from one saying Harvard mistreats women as "objects of lust whose intrusion into a contemplative society destroys both tranquility and intellectual life." I finally started distrusting our guise as equals, but I still couldn't see body-based inequity for the *sorrow* it brought me. When I graduated in '63 the college saw fit for the first time to promote women from Radcliffe to Harvard degrees. Since it now ranked all of us tops, I was solely to blame if my life fell short of LIFE.

I carried all this self-misgiving forward a few years later, into RA.

Because I owned an equal diploma, being female presented a problem I didn't yet have the word *sexism* for. After graduation I lived at a Harvard field station in Chiapas, where I raised delicate questions of land ownership, deeply grateful when one informant opened deeds of trust. But I didn't report to anyone that he always put his hand on my knees and then moved it up. No, I figured this was the price for bringing a foreign body into Mexico, asking about boundaries. Later in New York,

sharing a flat with my friend Adele and three other women, I heard
bitter stories of sexual harassment, date rape, back-alley procedures.
We thought we'd freed the body, but before legal contraception or
abortion or women's rights.

Six years later, as I rock a sleeping one-year-old, I'm struck by the
ways those unreported injuries prepared me to conceal RA. I remember
believing the body's problems ought to stay private, being so peculiar,
an idea I took from reading Flannery O'Connor. Diagnosed with "the
misery," as she called lupus (the first autoimmune disease I heard of),
she wrote, "I have never been anywhere but sick."

Since I had never been anywhere but well, I supposed that every
"misery" had its own antidote: cortisone for lupus, tranquilizers for
nerves, amphetamines for body fat, and fanfare estrogens for birth
control. I thought if misery ever happened to me—but why should
it?—I'd hide it till my pill-packed drugstore shooed it off.

For the time being I popped amphetamines to stay thin, harboring
a secret fear that my narrow body might be my older brother's in drag.
I'd watched him drop out of Harvard, take a Camel in one hand, a Coke
in the other, and gain a great many pounds. Just in case fatness was
fate in my family, my private journals narrowed down to the things
I ate. But when my brother and I talked, it was never about this. He
simply bullied me to agree with his certainties. By '65 he was a civil
rights activist, telling me to distrust the government, like all authority.
He complained that it segregated Medicare and handed out welfare
instead of healthcare—concerns that seemed remote to me at the time.
He defended his free choice of bad health and his civil right to keep
smoking and playing bridge for exercise.

Naturally our parents expected the straight and narrow from me.
In fact they expected nothing I couldn't tell them about. So I became
a sneak. I secretly left the country to visit a Latin American boyfriend
my parents weren't neutral about. Then I was found out and not let
off easy. My father railed at "lies which you try to cover with honeyed
phrases, laughing at us while you deceive." That needless note replaced
my natural love with something else: a guilty daughter's duty. After a
time I wrote back: "You are afraid about my life. Well, so am I, for god's
sake, *not knowing what pain I'm going to have*. Whatever happens, any
money from you I will pay back when I have a job."

It came down, absolutely, to a job. Or to the other female option.

My brother mentioned knowing a Jewish Harvard graduate I might like. "I haven't met John," I confided to my journal, "but am completely ready to fall in love because the externals of his life sound right." This reasoning couldn't end well, but when I did meet John, he made me laugh and took me skating and hiking, read me Max Beerbohm, played me Mozart, and then I dreamed: "Swimming in the sea where John kept searching for me—finally found me underwater, pitch black by then, did mouth-to-mouth rescue, and a tremendous gush came out of my lungs."

A few months later I jotted down "the way my heart jumped the first time he said *marriage*." And a little later: "I'd say offhand we'll live together this summer and get married next February." We did live together that summer and get married the next February, a joyous wedding on the day I turned twenty-five.

All through 1966 I tried to stay within a few feet of John, besotted by one body belonging to another—though mine was a swimmer's, swift and narrow, his tall and soccer formed. Privately I listed a few things I wanted to do with him: "teach, have children (optimally four), plus Peace Corps type thing. Possessions: dogs, no fish. And a harpsichord." Well, I did get to teach.

I also pulled up East Coast roots and transferred graduate work from Columbia to Stanford, for John's job. One day I slipped into a lecture of his and marveled that someone so at ease had fastened onto my anxious spirit for life. After the class I walked right into an antiwar protest, blown-up photos of blown-up bodies, and felt so alarmed I joined it and kept on joining. As violence pockmarked the coming presidential campaigns, I was also shaken for another reason. My brother was the chief software designer of the first electronic system reporting vote counts, so if anything bugged up the peace-versus-war results, he'd stand to blame.

All in all 1968 seemed a good time to quit the States. I was ready to write a dissertation in Chile, and John put in for a year's leave. One colleague queried him, "You're doing all that for the little woman?" Another asked, "Why don't you go to an important country?" meaning European. After this arrogance among the nicest liberals, a year in

Chile humbled us. Our friends there, working for Salvador Allende, half suspected us of being CIA. "What paranoia," I said to John at first. "CIA? In Chile?" Finally I was forced to cast off the myths I'd always counted on. Like "fair's fair."

These political wake-ups of the sixties had something to offer my private life too. They showed me how to recognize unfairness, such as signs that women, even well-trained ones, tended to fall behind. No one would rush to hire me if I went into child-bearing mode, and only my typist would skim my thesis for sure, whereas John's work on Chilean poet Pablo Neruda became a book that people would pay him to read. Offered coeducation, I was treated like a drain on male utilities. Handed an equal diploma, I was shamed by a female body. I was shown medical science, but no one like me doing it. I was urged to use brains *if* I used beauty too, to pursue a livelihood *if* love came first.

I made up my mind to change some of that.

En route from Chile to teach and do research in England, John and I visited my friend Adele in Tunisia and watched her work for social equality, as an equal, with her husband. We looked over our lives and our love, decided we'd divide all our tasks down the middle, knew we'd be delighted with a child, and started skipping birth control.

Pregnant in 1968, I ripened like a new idea. For my birthday, along with flowers, John gave me *Baby and Child Care*, a refreshed 1968 edition for the mother-to-be. I placed it right beside my own mother's dog-eared 1946 version and received the first shock of maternity. The new book repeated old passages as if social upheavals had skipped the home front. Dr. Spock, standing high for opposing the Vietnam war, was still advising: "Some mothers *have* to work to make a living. *Usually* their children turn out all right. . . . I wouldn't disagree if a mother felt strongly about it, provided she had an *ideal* arrangement for her children's care" (italics very much mine).

Into these words were poured mirages of nonworking, home-happy mothers and "ideal" childcare, which sent me straight to the women's movement. I suddenly couldn't do without it, having a baby to come and a thesis to finish and a job to search for. I even resented the female potential for "morning sickness" and informed John curtly, "Sickness just doesn't *agree* with me."

I saw myself as equal to any task—overturning past inequities, becoming a hands-on mother and an energetic earner and a share-alike partner. Nothing could hold this woman back. Nothing had the means of getting in her way.

Fatigue, 1971–74

Two years after the birth. "Listen, John," I say, hoisting our toddler from an unmade bed. "This is wearing me ragged." By now RA is penetrating every joint.

"I could do more," John says.

"Then you'd feel beat too."

So here we are, trapped by share-and-share-alike. It took two of us to conceive a baby, bring her through newborn jaundice and infant colic, raise her from crawling to toddling, and now one of us is a daily runner and the other a daily straggler. Just a few hours playing with Sarah and I'm readier than she is for a morning nap. Finally RA fatigue pushes me to a new idea: "All I want is subsidized on-site daycare, open all the time."

John bobs his head: that's good, dream on. Then he wiggles two fingers. "Hey, Sarah-Bear, you're almost two. And your mom's a Ph.D. today."

"I'm giving commencement a miss."

"Missing your doctorate?"

"Yep. The times we begged for a childcare center, Stanford just blinked."

"You're sure we're skipping it?" Pause. "Then it's OK if we split the day?" Meaning Sarah-care.

"Fine, fine."

So she's on my hands when a new motive for graduation dawns on me. Publicity. With John on a tennis court somewhere, not knowing the plan, I tank up a diaper bag and head for a degree, sans cap, sans gown.

Commencement day is a roaster, reminding me California is a desert with sprinklers. There's nowhere for my toddler to cool off. She's stuck squirming in my arms while we wait for our names to be called. In the line my friend Karen is nursing a newborn under her academic robes, and I see such gutsiness in mothers that I forget my aching shoulders, holding my little charge.

On her back I tape a sign—WHY CAN'T STANFORD SUPPORT CHILDCARE?—that gains appeal as Sarah chirps through the solemn ceremony. To occupy her mouth, I pull out chocolate bars, sludgy in the heat, until it's my turn to march across the podium. Seeing the poster child, the crowd takes the point and bursts into a roar. On that sound I float toward the dean to perform the doctoral maneuver—reach under the baby, take the diploma, and shake his hand. But when mine withdraws, it leaves his slick. And I alone know it's chocolate.

Marching offstage (the crowd still cheering), I'm bursting to move on. I call out to history graduates nearby, "Anyone know of a job?" One friend shouts back, "At Sonoma State. Part-time. Women's history."

Fine, except I do Latin America, and all I know about women's history is I need more childcare. Still, Sarah and I are stars for now, so I say, "Right. Who do I call?"

The next day I phone for an interview, and then John supplies meals on wheels while I work straight through the library's HQ call numbers, the women's history shelf—only a one-week read in 1971. The first book I open, Kate Millett's Sexual Politics, promises a "social revolution, quite unknown before in history." By the end of the week and the HQ shelf I believe that deposing men's power over women's bodies is where a revolution should start.

What began as tidbits to help me land a history job I'm gulping now as proteins. In the hiring interview I hear my voice say with energy, "Bias against women's bodies is the key to inequality," and I marvel at the chanciness that turns me toward female physiques. My new purpose isn't to depose any male powers I make use of. It's to expose a crucial insight: the uncertain state of every woman's body in a world men run.

When I get the part-time job at Sonoma State, north of San Francisco, I'm astonished by students creating health collectives, self-healing groups, childcare co-ops—nothing my fine schools gave any lessons in—and I step up. In a family experiment John, moves to Sonoma for my job, and while I teach, he carries Sarah on his shoulders for long rural hikes. In another experiment, for final exams, I'm seen

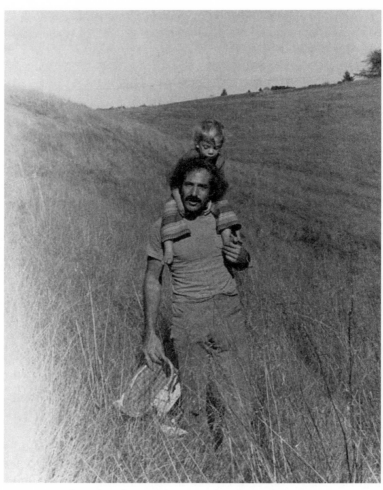

John and Sarah in Sonoma, 1971. Photo by Martha Sommer.

taping shelf paper over the floor so students can write answers in graf-fiti. As I grade on hands and knees (a painful exercise I should avoid), the faculty splits over rehiring me. Their meeting runs long, and before they vote no, I dial (on their nickel) every other Bay Area college. Are you intending to offer a class in women's history?

"Not *yet*," most colleges laugh. "Sure," says San Francisco State, adding, "You'd have to teach Latin America too." My field!

Now I need a strategy for full-time teaching with full-time RA, and what I come up with is: shh! About many issues I'll rage and complain and carry posters. But about my disease I keep quiet.

My doctor also treats it quietly, as any 1970s rheumatologist would. He waits to see if twenty aspirin a day calm it. No? Then he raises me one level on the treatment slope, to strong antimalarials that lower the fever between bones.

"But why do joints get so hot?" I ask.

"It's the body reacting to injury," he explains, "by passing blood through the vessel walls into the tissues, bringing redness and swelling and heat and pain."

"What injury?" I want to know, but I won't bring myself to ask if I somehow inflicted it. I'm afraid of an answer.

"Inflammation shows up first in the synovial tissue," says Dr. B.

"Right." I've looked up *synovial*, being a teacher and all: it's a membrane around an ovum-like, egg-like joint. It looks like the skim on tapioca pudding. Inflamed synovial tissues bulge with immune cells slipping from the bloodstream, causing pain.

"And one indicator of active disease is your rheumatoid factor—"

"Right." This one I haven't looked up.

"It's an autoantibody inside the joints of almost everyone with RA. It binds to another antibody, creating an autoimmune reaction that triggers inflammation." He sits down, glad to be talking science.

I don't know the workings of these words—*antibody, autoimmune, inflammation*—and don't want to. What I get from this: I'm to take drugs as if I have malaria. I'm to send my steamy joints on safari, slipping exotic pills into my homely medicine cabinet, along with the calamine and Band-Aids, the Nivea crème, the Bayer.

The first little discovery I allow myself, now that my treatment's getting serious, is that rheumatologists build a pyramid of care, trying everything gradually, one tier at a time. So far I've stayed near the base, since doctors prescribe aspirin until they see physical damage. So far I've envisioned a disease quick to hurt but slow to destroy, thinking "aspirin's strong enough" and not guessing that inflammation has been cracking into my joints.

My doctor's routine moves on. "Let's go to the knees. Your right knee's a little stiff."

"Mmhm."

"How're your elbows feeling?"

"Mmf."

My second discovery about arthritis: language isn't up to it. To show the doctor where it hurts, I press a painful finger on an inflamed shoulder, but the double sting of touching and being touched is indescribable.

"A little tender here?" He's squeezing the shoulder. "A little warm too?" Empathic words for pain he doesn't endure. Then he flips through the chart, asks about my work, and, astonishingly, records what he sees in me—namely, a caretaking sort of patient, pulling herself through fatigue: "She feels that she lacks energy but she is really one of the most incredibly energetic people I know. She is up around 6:30 a.m., goes to the City for 14 hours a day, works teaching four different classes at S.F. State, then she returns to take care of her house, her daughter. In the meantime she sandwiches in political activities, activities for Amnesty International, and a variety of other organizations."

Then he says, almost done, "How's Arthur?"

"You mean John? My husband?"

"Arthur."

"Arthur who?"

"Arthur-itis."

From a rheumatologist I hear this, so I laugh.

I laugh too when Sarah holds up five fingers and says "cinco" because we're in Mexico for the summer. It's the age she has reached—and so, it seems, has RA. That they sprang to life together is not something I stress, in case the charge for my condition would fall on her. In the last years I've simply focused on the basics: that it's here to stay, that it delivers fatigue, demands solutions, moves faster than easy treatments. No new insight comes along for awhile, until I'm staying in a Mexican village, eating tortillas at every meal. Then I discover that most tortillas come off a conveyor belt because women weary of hand work demanded a mechanized shop, and this brought wiring to the village. I'm seeing a secret source of human progress: women's joint complaints.

For the first time I think maybe aching joints serve some larger design. This strikes me again in the village church when my eye catches handmade votive paintings. *Votive* must come from *votum*, "vow," a word I dredge up from high school Latin. The tiny painted figures vow devotion to a saint in case the sufferer is cured. On the off-chance I can bargain too—I'll take RA if some larger good comes of it—I vow selfless devotion to my loved ones. Only my 1974 diary knows this comes hard:

> After dinner I say: "Sarah, my friend, it's eight o'clock." She says back, "That isn't interesting." To make it interesting, I bet she's going to demand someday, "What were you chasing so hard that you weren't more with me?" I'll have to say, I couldn't do it all, with RA, so I became your mother at work. Not *my* mother at home.
>
> Later at night John falls asleep, all lean and brown against a white sheet. He dreams he's waking to tell me his dream but I get impatient. Then he wakes and tells me his dream and I get impatient. I'm too self-involved—with a stiff wrist, an ankle that feels hammered, a devilish elbow.

Back home my doctor is now suggesting elbow surgery, which sparks an Elizabeth Cady Stanton response. I tell Sarah at bedtime that Stanton's baby had a bent collarbone, and the doctor's brace caused pain, so this founding suffragist "made a sling out of diapers, fixed the bone, and never accepted the word of any man again."

I'm thrilled a day later to hear Sarah say "Stanton" to a preschool friend.

"Who's that?" he asks.

"Oh," my daughter says, "she's the lady who invented diapers."

I laugh here too, knowing I'm not the lady to invent anything or heal any bone. I'm the sort to double the antimalarials and top off my twenty aspirin with a few more. Sarah watches me pop pills with the canny eyes of a five-year-old. Then something happens that shows arthritis can damage even her.

One day, left alone, she gets a notion to copy her mom by emptying a hidden bottle of medication into her mouth, then secretly replaces the pills with raisins. Hours go by before we come on the raisins and rush to Emergency to have her stomach pumped. It's a grave wait to make

sure she wasn't poisoned by arthritis remedies. After that we hide the
sealed bottle on a higher shelf and tell her to stay out of the pills. But
she is a social climber, a monkey-doer, and looks right back as if to say,
You mean stay out of the raisins.

This time my silent vow is specific: I'll pay attention to others' health.
So the next event comes as a shock:

> Listening to Pete Seeger singing "Abi Yoyo" Sarah says, "I
> can't hear the 'Yoyo.'" The doctor pronounces neither
> ear working right—a common infection but a serious
> case. How am I (of all people) supposed to believe a se-
> rious case goes away? I'm scared for her. And ashamed
> of not noticing the signs. At the same time John's worry-
> ing he'll have his father's heart disease, and exercising
> like a zealot.
>
> My 33rd birthday passes with my knee shooting at me,
> my elbow touchy, my tongue sharp. Finally Sarah says
> to me: "I know a pear that got so angry it died into a
> raisin."

I'm not dying into a raisin yet. But I'm requesting a family exemp-
tion, having paid some dues with arthritis.

I know it's not dues that eventually bring back Sarah's hearing, it's
antibiotics tubed into her ears. But I wouldn't mind making a votive
painting anyway. It would show an Angel of Anatomy with huge wings,
looking helpful and maybe vengeful, hovering near my home. Like the
angel that razed Pharaoh's tribe but passed over Israelite slaves, my
invented figure goes about distributing sickness or safety. The Angel
of Anatomy caps pill bottles and unclogs ears, waives inherited heart
disease, beats away cancer because I've already done my share with
RA—in other words passes over *everything* in order to swoop down on
my stiffened joints.

It's taken five years to stumble on a useful image for my trouble. If
it's a long disease I'm stuck with, then let it be a decoy.

Promises, 1975–76

"Let my people go," we're singing at our Passover table.

To be let go for awhile doesn't seem too much to ask of this ritual of liberation. After seven lean years with RA I'm calling on a Passover promise: seven seasons in bondage, the next one free.

Freedom is like a promised land, and John wants it literal: we should spend next year in Jerusalem. To join him there I take Sarah across ten time zones on an El Al plane where I keep repeating my one word of Hebrew, "Shalom." Right after landing, when I dawdle in my seat, a stewardess calls, "Lama?" and I wheel around, shocked to know another word, from singing Bach's St. *Matthew Passion*. The word *why*? Why hast thou forsaken me?

From that day whatever I learn has to do with the subject of suffering, that is, the smallness of my own and my fellow-feeling for others' pain. I'm thinking of my great-grandfather, who took a wretched voyage here in 1882, with the famous first fourteen Russian Jewish settlers, and distinguished himself by dying right away. I enter Israel under his omen (mind your health) and St. Matthew's, whose gospel promises to punish Jewish children forever. *Lama?* Why Jewish children? It's only a year since Egypt, Syria, Jordan, and Iraq attacked Israel on Yom Kippur, and most Israeli women my age have at least one child on patrol. In Israel it's only fair for me to feel pained. Arthritis serves for some of that.

At a musical party one night I discover another way to think about suffering. From a shelf I pull out a book of paintings by Charlotte Salomon, a German Jewish artist who had just finished a thousand brilliant images of her life when the Nazis deported her, at age twenty-six. Amazed and horrified, I turn toward the music in the next room, a soprano performing Mozart's *Exsultate, Jubilate*, a soaring song I instantly want to know by heart. I want to rise above peril and create

something transcendent, as Charlotte Salomon did. I want to learn
singing. While everyone listens to dreadful news, my ear will tune to
"Exult, Rejoice."

I sign up for lessons with the soprano. I open my throat. After four
months my voice box cracks.

By this point I can't help catching the pattern with RA. Try something
new? Strain something more. Soreness of voice is what I bring home
from Israel. I also bring slides of Charlotte Salomon paintings that I
show to my students and later to high schools and churches. Audiences
always call out, Why haven't we heard of her? What was her life like?
And I say, "I'll go find out," because I don't understand that the Nazis
meant to erase every memory of Jews.

I still think loss can't be in full—not loss of voice, at least. But then
a specialist writes in my chart: "This patient is worried about having to
teach school and afraid she might injure her voice or lose it. Comment:
Probably the quality will not improve."

It doesn't. But suddenly the rest of me goes into remission. It's a
word I've read in the Christian Bible, where the Lord grants remission
of sins. But true to pattern in chronic diseases, it's only a parole—which
might last weeks or years, my doctor says—while the body sends back
symptoms.

To me remission means the freedom to skip paraffin dips, to splash
in the Stanford swimming pool with Sarah, to slice my way down the
lanes. In the evenings remission means hours I can give to articles and
deadlines. It's my time to win tenure, to rush to my papers as soon as
Sarah's asleep. This greatly impresses my desk.

Like everyone with a chronic condition I reach the stage of pretending
it's remitted for good. I even ask John, "If we could share RA between
us"—if the Angel of Anatomy could throw a switch—"would we?"

John nods his head. Before he says yes, I take out a notebook and
start writing, "Tasks to Share, 1976." His include half of the childcare
and the five carpools we organize, plus getting babysitters and cleaning
the garage (every few years). Mine feature an item called "coordination
of the schedule," plus the other half of childcare and carpools and
handling lousy joints. "All our colleagues manage better," I complain,

"having wives." I read Arlie Hochschild's "Inside the Clockwork of Male Careers," which moves me to tears by exposing women's burden of working and caring for kids and pitching in everywhere unpaid. In our household even slicing tasks down the middle floors me, with a disease added on top.

John says, "Why don't we each do whatever we can?"

"I wouldn't know where to stop."

Long pause. "What's your doctor say?"

That afternoon in his office I listen to Dr. B. dictate: "Mary continues to work harder than she should and is more tired than she should be."

Remission hasn't done away with fatigue. For almost a decade I've been tired and keeping quiet about it. What matters to me actively is the women's movement and any other cause I beat my anger into. What also matters to me is looking less good than I did before RA. In a journal I scribble: "Depressing news from the doctor today about enlarged lymphs, salivary, throat. My first impulse: buy an enormous cheeseburger. My second impulse: have a real triumph by not buying a cheeseburger." Then I notice I react to arthritis by taking false control.

The "depressing news" concerns anemic blood cells and swollen glands that didn't get word of remission, forcing me to grasp what's meant by *systemic disease*. I'm tempted to take these words to a women's group I've joined, but from the start a member says, "What we share should be political."

"Should we only complain of abuses?" I ask. No one speaks. I decide I can't mention my joints—not a women's issue, apparently, though plenty of medical problems are. We circulate hand to hand the 1976 manual *Our Bodies, Ourselves*. From this brave new source I'm learning that Our Bodies have hot flashes and sexually transmitted diseases and cervical cancer—but never joints. I come across arthritis only once, as a possible by-product of gonorrhea.

"Am I that odd?" I ask my doctor one day.

"Let's see, you're thirty-five, when RA is the most common."

Common does describe arthritis. I find brochures saying that its hundred forms, along with other musculoskeletal disorders, are the nation's leading cause of disability. But they're a problem with no name in a movement that now names everything, from "date rape" to "pro-choice," a movement that creates shelters, bookstores, clinics—maybe not as brassy as Black Power and antiwar resistance but tackling injustice every day. It's as if joints have no bearing on rights, as if some woman with RA can forget she's insurable as some man's wife, can ignore the strains in share-alike, the best deal she'll get. Suddenly I don't know where to turn if not to feminism. And I can't mention this to my women's group.

I don't even mention to myself what arthritis has done to my toes. Now they're drifting sideways, five to starboard, five to port, which I forget in planning a remission trip, backpacking near Yosemite. But something unforeseen happens there, adding the word *hobbled* to recent acquisitions like *systemic*. The trip starts with putting Sarah on a camp bus, her seven-year-old face so small the windowsill cuts across her chin. "We could take her home," John says, but we stand there until I say, "Everyone likes camp," remembering no such thing. Slowly we inch backward toward our car.

That evening on a trail I marvel at my sturdy knees, two of the seven wonders of the world, but my feet keep stumbling on a rock and a hard place. "Let's stop and sleep outside," I finally say. Late that night I wake to find a great upstanding bear no further from my feet than my feet are from my head.

I poke John, and we tumble into the tent, pulling a nylon flap between ourselves and that wildness. "Run?" I ask frantically, as if my drifting toes could sprint.

"Now?"

"You decide."

"I can't," John says.

"You *decide*."

And there it is, an end to equality. The man must make the plan. But he won't, so we hold each other till daylight, then stare at tracks around and around the tent.

Two nights later the bear litters a new campsite with our food. "John, we've got nothing left to eat."

"Well, neither does the bear," says John and pulls me, weak and faltering, to the trailhead. We descend to a store, buy quick-calorie chocolate and Cheez Whiz, then drive to meet the camp bus, coated with kids' food. When Sarah scampers over and takes us in a tangly hug (she calls it a "love-bunch"), a delight comes over me, a message I know will keep repeating: she's making it on her own.

My joints can't do that anymore, even to save their lives.

I feel hobbled now, when I should be hitting my stride. I'm a full-time tenured teacher whose active parts are eroding, cartilage vanishing and muscles loosening. That's why my toes are drifting, the doctor says— and I must advance up the treatment pyramid. I say, "Give me time," like months and months.

But I realize my best defenses so far (delay and deny) are costing me some joints. Finally, after years of low-tier aspirin and antimalarials, I rise to a venerable remedy for RA: gold. In my clinic one day I learn that gold interferes with overachievers in my bloodstream—lymphocytes that attack infection and antibodies that neutralize foreign-looking proteins. As a bonus the brilliant metal lands me a place "on the rand," which is not the South African goldfield I imagine but a Rolodex file of recurrent patients. On the rand my name is known, my vein is known. While a technician each week coaxes blood from my scarred vessels, testing for gold-degraded kidneys, I take this lying down and scotch all hopes I used to have about being brave.

After the blood test I mince toward the gold injection. Because a dense metal enters the body grudgingly, the nurse punches in a kind of horse shot. "Hang on. This will sting."

I distract myself, intoning, Worth my weight in gold.

"All done."

But I'm not done at all. Driving away after the shot, I see there's no going back to before. I remember speeding past vegetable stands on this Palo Alto road and shops where I could get a vacuum fixed. The shift to fancy franchises looks like progress, but my eye catches the closeouts. My joints match my neighborhood, gilded but gone fragile.

By the time I pull up to a swimming pool near home, I've made a discovery: that the promise in a metaphor—this year in pain, next year free—has sent me across the world, lifted my voice to soprano, opened the gates of remission, raised my consciousness in groups, pitted my body against wilderness, saturated my bloodstream with gold, convinced me with the Beatles it's getting better all the time, while the truth is: it's getting worse.

At Passover I believed bondage couldn't last. Now I realize what doesn't last: remission. Seven years into RA I backstroke painfully up and down the pool, with no inkling how I'll get to go forward again.

Alternatives, 1979

Three years later whenever John asks, after a long day, "Swim with me?" I shake my head. I have to admit my sweet remission has vanished, lingering no more than a year. Sarah has turned ten, and my old premarriage desire—"children (optimally four)"—seems cruelly out of bounds. But I still have a longing for optimally two, so once in awhile John and I weigh the alternatives. I say, "I'm not sure it's possible." He sits down while I take a breath to add, "Antimalarials and gold would overdose a fetus . . . even if we're ready, you know, for a baby again."

For hours we turn the question over, but it's beyond us. Without pills for nine months would I collapse, or would alternative treatments steady me till another child? Then would my joints be able to deal with taking care of one? Finally I remember a trick of my parents, who never lazed around in their personal lives if they could expose segregated housing or steelworker wages. They passed to me their fact-finding drive and their dissent, which could help now: I'm foundering in my condition and need a different take on it.

That's how I come to Susan Sontag's *Illness as Metaphor*, a dissenting 1978 book claiming that the early seventies distorted cancer into a metaphor (John Dean: "we have a cancer within—close to the presidency") and that this misuse reflected anxiety about an uncontrolled economy. Suddenly I'm able to see arthritis as a metaphor for more recent years: it's the sluggish aftermath of growth, the frazzling of energy since the '73 oil crisis. It stands for recession, as in "the economy moves at arthritic speed." No wonder it's abhorred: incurable, unspeakable, recessionary.

Until reading Sontag, or Ivan Illich's 1976 *Medical Nemesis*, I do not realize that recession doubles the patients on Medicare and Medicaid, that medicine can add to the suffering it's supposed to fix, or that nonurgent operations end the lives of twelve thousand people yearly—

more civilians dying on nearby gurneys than U.S. soldiers in Vietnam. I do not realize the "failure of heroic medicine to cure" till reading Regina Morantz. But I do know it's perilous to start doubting medicine's claim of helping bodies and improving lives. It would throw me into the hands of alternative healers. And what if I doubt these too?

This question leads to the next one, as I make my commute after teaching: what do I want now?

I want to blame my stinking joints on . . . John. OK, this is promising, but don't ride the brake.

I also want to be worthy of—watch that station wagon on the left—worthy of mothering again. But suppose a tiny baby is a sinker on my body.

I better get off the freeway at Sand Hill Road before the after-school program closes. "How was school?" I ask as Sarah jumps in the car.

"Fine."

"After-school?"

"Fine."

"How was the lunch John made you?"

"Fine."

"Oh honey, I hope it's all true, all fine."

At home I empty her lunchbox, with one crescent bitten from the whole-wheat-and-tofu sandwich, then realize I've been wanting to answer "Fine" too for quite some time. In the air of the seventies there's faith that people will do fine with alternative medicine, fine with Chinese remedies now that diplomatic lines are open, fine with the organic sandwiches that Sarah leaves in the lunchbox. Even RA patients do fine on their own, if a third of them go into remission whether treated by doctors or not.

But I'm not in that third. By now I've tried and failed to get relief from acupressure, macrobiotic and high-protein diets, massage, self-hypnosis—every decent alternative the seventies has on offer—and I'm wary of the sting in other self-treatments. Arthritis consumers are shelling out $950 million on unproven remedies: copper bracelets circle fifty million wrists at $35 per arm; for every dollar going to arthritis research, $25 heads toward "mistreatment," as I read one day in *Consumer Reports*. The members of my slow-moving subgroup—and here's an irony for you—are the nation's speediest spenders on "do-it-yourself" cures.

The next day I'm in Stanford Library, handling the do-it-yourself book of 1979, *Anatomy of an Illness*, in which Norman Cousins masters a severe rheumatic attack by rejecting a "cycle of fear, depression, and panic," by "bucking the odds." His self-treatment: laughter, because it seems to "reduce inflammation in my joints." I like the cut of his cure. Why don't I just buck the odds? Then I remember that his ailment came from exposure to jet fuel, while mine lives deep in immune cells where ignorant armies clash by night.

It's Cousins's view of pain that finally throws me off. He blames "promiscuous use" of painkillers for creating "psychological cripples and chronic ailers." Promiscuous and cripples? I have to block those metaphors with hands that can't hold the hardback between them, with smoldering shoulders that hurt when I laugh. "Pain-killing turns people into unfeeling spectators of their own decaying selves," writes Ivan Illich. Uh, I'm afraid it's pain that does that. I shove the books back on the shelf, then stop and admit they've taught me lessons anyway—that I need to read about health to make decisions for my life, that I can't swallow heroic medicine whole and can't fall for alternatives either, and that I'm ready to try *something* new.

I try imagining my hard-working grandma with arthritis, which no one in my family ever had. She'd have called on public health in the 1920s, and they'd have said, "REST," and she'd have said, "On the *bed?*" Later, if her daughter Anne, my mother, had suffered arthritis, which she didn't, her doctor in the 1930s would have suggested, once again, REST. Even today, I realize, most arthritic joints are told to go easy, and that's about that.

But now there's a turnabout in treatment starting a mile from where I'm strenuously resting. Dr. James Fries, director of Stanford's Arthritis Clinic, claims that every single joint will profit from exercise. His popular 1979 book, *Arthritis: A Comprehensive Guide*, says exercise helps joints by squeezing waste products out of cartilage (which is three-fourths water and compresses like a sponge), then sucking back joint fluid, nutrients, and oxygen. Dr. Fries cautions that rheumatoid arthritis ("the most destructive kind of arthritis known") causes "erosions of the bone itself, rupture of tendons, and slippage of the joints" and makes most sports (except swimming or walking) a danger. Still, if exercise can "fight anxiety and depression," it tucks nicely into the view that upbeat moods heal illnesses. There's also news of mutual-aid groups like the National Black Women's Health Project, or Stanford-run support groups helping thousands of arthritis patients exercise so that they live in less pain and actually drop some disability. This sounds so good I might take up self-help or exercise. Then pregnancy.

At the end of a decade that assures me, wrongly, any health dilemma can be dealt with, my doctor once again reviews the dilemma he calls "the desirability of her getting pregnant vs. the desirability of taking gold."

Of those two choices I chose gold—actually pain chose it for me. But now I'm open to any reason to reverse. Dr. B. says, "If you want a baby—"

"I think so."

"What's your husband say?"

"That it's exhausting with RA, two jobs, shared childcare . . ."

"If you want a baby, stop the gold."

"I want a baby being *well*."

"You'll feel better during pregnancy. Women with RA usually do."

This is such good news I decide not to know what happens afterward. Soon I start tugging on John. Suppose I go without gold? Suppose we rouse our energies for another child? John says it's finally up to me.

Once I'm gold free and pregnant, my body slips into charmed remission again. I'm springing around the neighborhood, thinking health thoughts that aren't about joints. Thinking how my obstetrician says I'm a natural for pregnancy, and that's true: I'm overjoyed with it. I'm also a natural for women's choice, which he doesn't see when declaring he "won't do Roe v. Wades."

Still, I like his sharing his new technology with me, offering a pair of earphones to track a fetal heart. "Hear that?"

"No."

"Listen again. Hear it?"

"YES."

How astonishing. Each visit for months I strap on the earphones, and the heart's *there* again, the thrilling autonomous thump.

I feel so good I need to look good too and go off to a spa so I'll end up after birth as slim as before pregnancy. I soak in a hot tub (no warnings that pregnant women shouldn't) and three days later, at a Passover Seder, feel a very slight trickle on my leg.

"Doesn't sound too serious," the obstetrician says on the phone. "Come tomorrow around ten."

Right at ten I'm on the examining table, strapping on the earphones for the heartbeat. Nothing there. I do *not* need to not hear that.

The doctor orders, "Bear down, Mary! Push," and I deliver: a late-fifth-month miscarriage, technically a stillbirth, what the doctor calls a "baby boy!"

John glances at my jammed-shut eyes and on the next beat says, "Don't you mean fetus?"—words that matter a good deal, even at that moment, words at war. I never again want a doctor who does miscarriages but refuses abortions, who would call this stricken thing a "baby boy!" And I never again want to get intimate with *anything* perishing inside my skin.

Pregnant one week and not the next, I hear my colleagues, to a man, assure me I'll be pregnant again, but all I see is a perfect sphere of loss. Then a colleague who's hardly noticed me looks straight in my eyes and says the one true thing: "This is heartbreaking."

Heartbreaking to follow pregnancy, again, with pain. This is the loss that finally assembles ten years of losses, tangling them into one undeniable knot. On the sofa between John and Sarah I reach for that knot, visible to no one else. In one decade I've lost my guarantee of good health, lost fluidity, lost ease in the physical acts of parenting, lost a fair practice of equal tasks, lost nouns like *energy* and *swiftness*, lost my lifelong singing voice and even a speaking voice free of crackles and pops, lost my elbow grease for vacuuming and yard work and tearing full speed down a swimming lane, lost any assurance I could run from threats, lost my trust in feminists to name my woes, lost my reliance on medicine and also on alternatives, lost my remission, lost my pregnancy. Amid all the losses what can never be found again is my old sense that each loss must be a fluke.

Each one is knotted in. For this is RA, this is chronic, this has design.

I try to focus on my terrific child and partner and job. Look how I've come through the decade—with tenure, with essays on revolution and on feminism, with phone messages from friends, with care for their problems, with adventures watching our fourth-grader. Look at her swimming the crawl with a flutter kick to die for. Or racing down the soccer field with energy enough to yell as she passes the bench, "What's for snack?" And look at her sitting beside John and unrolling her day, as I ask them to tell me about it, then tell me more. Here's John handing me a peeled carrot, saying "You're beautiful," as he looks at my tight-ribbed sweater and newly narrow waist. Here's Sarah trying out tunes on her new flute. And here's a wingbeat passing over, the Angel of Anatomy, my votive figure, my imagined tribune, announcing: I give you all of the above, but I also take away.

Some months later, by good fortune, I'm expecting again—thrilled, wary, skeptical, thinking no one congratulating me understands my disease.

Well, do I? Most days arthritis just takes me over, puts me down to nap. I've never yet stood back to question how it's *working*. I've detested it too much to give it features and causes, a meaning in the world. But now that a new baby's coming, I've got to get wise to it. I call this out, banging the kitchen table, surprising Sarah and John.

And soon enough I get wise to the worst part about it.

II. Getting Wise

> The problem, unstated till now, is how
> to live in a damaged body
> in a world where pain is meant
> to be gagged.

Adrienne Rich,
The Fact of a Doorframe

Inflammation, 1980–84

Pain, the long and short of it. Not the endless ache of RA but the sharp contractions of my second childbirth make me pant like a sick dog and scream for a Cesarean. Then abruptly the pain—I can't believe this—is swished away. A baby emerges and grabs air. John's knees fold as he whispers "My guy" and "Sweet feet" and for hours calms the tiny item with a syllable, a rhyme, a word, a rhyme.

By the next morning we go home and spend the day sliding over the bedroom rug, chasing a shaft of low December sun with the baby on our chests. Coiled in a blanket nearby, Sarah watches hour by hour. The baby is so tranquil. Quieter the next day. What luck.

Then we go back to the ward for a checkup and discover why he never cries.

He's full of jaundice. Before I can think "Please not again!" our baby's in intensive care, bound to repeat Sarah's bout with jaundice twelve years before. At least it's more treatable since Sarah's day— since a nurse noticed that newborns near the ward windows recovered quickly, and a simple ultraviolet cure came into being.

For three days I stand by the baby's ultraviolet incubator, watching his misery, feeling my joints grow achy, and then, whoosh, up come wildfire flares. Heavy-handed, I fold him in a blanket as the nurse advises, "Give his body lots of sunlight to keep the jaundice down." So I carry him toward an unshaded fountain near the hospital and unwrap his blanket with stiffened hands.

A woman nearby sees me expose the baby to the winter air, steps up, and warns, "I'll report you."

"No. Really. We just have jaundice."

We.

Back home I talk to "Alek," named for John's Russian cousin Aleksandr, now in Siberian prison, and for Eleck, my dad. "Alek, little bupper, you're the best. But why'd you have to get jaundice?" And why'd I have to get white-hot flareups now, recalling the sudden inflammation after Sarah? A brand-new suspicion arrives—that the babies and I grew *allergic* to one another before birth, resulting in jaundice for them, joint pain for me. Twelve years into the disease, it's the first new thought I've had about its cause.

I call my family and close friends to say, "Alek's home, and I've never been happier in my life." Not a peep about the flareup. Quietly I search for "jaundice" in Dr. Spock's baby-care book, knowing my own mom asked Ben Spock in person about my newborn health, both of them working with children in Pittsburgh. Now that I'm the one seeking his advice, he only says jaundice "should be reported to the doctor" and implies, Put your worries away.

I turn to the new preface of the world-famous manual I used for Sarah in '69. The "main reason" Spock gives for this 1976 revision of *Baby and Child Care*: "to eliminate the sexist biases of the sort that helped create and perpetuate discrimination against girls and women. . . . I always assumed that the parent taking the greater share of the care of young children (and of the home) would be the mother."

He's saying he always assumed wrong. He's joining a cultural shift so profound I can finally let up. This time I won't have to fight an equity battle for basic childcare. But I confess to my diary that I'm unsettled:

> March '81.Taking care of an infant, I'm becoming just what a feminist shouldn't be—passionately focused on a baby of one's own. John says, nonsense, that I'm *always* talking about the casualties at Verdun.
> On a morning walk, Alek gets scratched by branches. My heart rushes out to him and we gratefully nurse. Then at three a.m. he starts crying. I grab Spock who's very calm: "Let him fuss 20 or 30 minutes." I'm counting. He screams two hundred seventy-three times.

At least the jaundice is gone and my flareup is cooling, so maybe I wasn't crazy to have another baby, along with RA. I'm about to keep the disease to myself again when a work trip abroad shows me how new-fashioned my secrecy is.

In '81 we leave California to spend four months wrapping the baby in snowsuits for what's known as English spring. Outside Taplow village, where we live, I sometimes walk near the Juvenile Rheumatism Center, famous since its founding in 1947 for helping children struck by excruciating juvenile rheumatoid arthritis, also called Still's disease. These children sometimes have twenty-five surgeries by adulthood and wear metal plates between their bones. I cry in pity and fear, then push Alek's stroller swiftly past. Note to Angel of Anatomy: Take my joints if you want, so long as you leave his alone.

At half a year this baby likes to return what's given. When he returns his latest meal into the pews of Taplow church, a woman across the aisle says, "Oh dear, he's being sick" (British for spitting up). I lift a burning shoulder in apology, and as we slip out though the nave, it strikes me that "being sick" takes such varied cultural meanings I might use my time outside my country to look into a few of them.

I find some social histories in the library, spread them on the window seat, and go so far as to learn that Romans two thousand years ago were dealing openly with my disease. While balancing Alek on one knee, I discover Celsus, a first-century physician who named four cardinal signs that point to inflammation:

> *calor*
> *rubor*
> *dolor*
> *turgor*

There's no problem translating the first three, but I'm stuck on *turgor*, and fetching back to high school Latin doesn't help. *Calor*, *rubor*, and *dolor*—heat, redness, and pain—appear when blood vessels dilate, inflamed cells leak into tissues, swell the skin hot and powder pink. These Latin words are so visual I'm drawn to see more, go somewhere Roman.

We decide to travel to Bath, where Roman legions found an answer to bone-aching British spring, making me look on them with new respect. They fused their healer Minerva with the local goddess Sul, to found Aquae Sulis, Waters of Sul, a multiplex of hot springs, clinics, and fleshpots. My eyes fill with heartfelt if freezing tears at their spacious thermal pools, their lubrications for the likes of joints.

Wandering Bath, my spirits also lift at the Enlightenment, which opened the world's first clinic devoted solely to the ancestors of my arthritis. I learn that patients arrived at "the Min," the great Royal Mineral Water Hospital of 1742, with joints so jackknifed they doubled over to walk and looked at the world backward through their legs. In one painting at the Min bewigged physicians carefully examine a worker's puffed, immobile hands (while his wife and child wait their turn), and my hands feel the gentle, genteel touch. That's when I recall the meaning of *turgor*. Stiffness, of course.

I know stiffness starts in the synovial fluid. Now it cheers me to read that *synovial* was a sixteenth-century coinage of Theophrastus Bombastus von Hohenheim, known as Paracelsus, meaning "smarter than Celsus," the Roman physician who named the four signs of inflammation. In Paracelsus's contempt for other physicians ("every little hair on my neck knows more than you . . . and my beard has more experience than all your high colleges") I imagine synovial fluid swelling with bombast and blocking the body's articulation until it can't express how fast a person like me wants to go.

Moving slowly around the city, I see the atrocities of inflammation that drew patients here for centuries. Bath's early clientele spent months in the waters. Later rheumatics tried high-dose gold injections (causing kidneys to fail), bone-shaving operations (leaving painful limps), organ-removing surgery (in case infections caused arthritis), spinal radiation (inviting leukemia), plaster casts (making muscles atrophy), finger amputation. Suddenly my antimalarials slide down like Devonshire cream. I feel a gratitude new to me, that I'm not a wretched rheumatic at the Min.

Later that day, threading through Bath's meeting rooms built for Jane Austen's world, I'm stunned by their sociability. "Look how aches and pains brought society here," I say to John. "In *Sense and Sensibility* Austen calls rheumatism 'the commonest infirmity of declining life.' In *Persuasion* people openly plan to 'come to Bath on that account.' So I've had it with modern furtiveness. Those thermal baths the Romans built, they're *enormous*. Like Austen's Pump Room and the Min. They were social investments in caring and cure."

The next morning, during a predawn attack against my joints, I decide any society ignoring *calor*, *rubor*, *dolor*, and *turgor* isn't Roman enough for me. Here in Europe a state or labor union would stand me to treatments at modern versions of Bath, but at home, with Ronald Reagan in office, fat chance of broader health funding, which requires an Enlightenment ideal of public good, if not a pantheist belief in healing. No, arthritis wasn't always private and isolating, and it doesn't have to be.

Dolor and calor shaped the lives of many others I can learn from. Before leaving Europe we travel to an Amsterdam exhibit of Charlotte Salomon, whose paintings from the 1940s, when she was hiding from the Nazis, tell the sorrowful story of living in a house of suicides. At twenty-three she learned that eight relatives had killed themselves, and had to ask "the question: whether to take her own life or to undertake something eccentric and mad," a life story in art. Inside my passport I fold a note saying, "If RA causes too much pain and inflammation, I'll need to keep the same question open."

Back at home I give a public talk on Charlotte Salomon where I meet a distant relative of John's. Aunt Ruth has a seventy-year-old wit along with thirty-year-old pain from RA. Commenting on suicides in Charlotte Salomon's family, she confesses to such crippling flareups she once asked her children: Would they understand if she simply had to take her life? "The question" posed by Salomon keeps company with my disease.

I come home from the talk fearing that flareups could take me from all that is good here—John at his desk, Alek banging a Fisher-Price xylophone, and Sarah saying, "He's so innocent, he doesn't know there's war and pollution and nuclear bombs. He only knows that he's completely loved." I rush to set this down in my diary, along with my own entry: "We don't get happiness and peace, only minutes of purity inside a deluge." It seems inflammation leads to more kinds of ruin than I'd imagined, from Roman calor to another Latin word, suicide, and the prospect of killing the pain. Then I come pretty close to consumption by calor myself.

It happens when John's mother dies of Alzheimer's, after forgetting what language is for, then family, then food. On the day of her death the Angel of Anatomy sends me warnings: Don't leave Alek with a sitter and risk flying through storms from San Francisco to New York for her

funeral. She's just orphaned her son, and that's what could happen to
your son.

John goes to the funeral, I stay safe at home and then not so safe. On
a biting December night I place a workman's light bulb under the hood
of our car so I can drive it to school for the last exam of 1984. Before bed
I notice the bulb's out, toss it behind the car. Late at night it toggles on
and heats some rags nearby. While we're sleeping a slow burn starts,
and soon the whole garage is blazing. I wake to find two men trying
to force their way in my door and finally realize they're shouting, "Get
out! Fire!" Before I can move, fifteen-year-old Sarah has grabbed Alek
from his crib and hurtled past me to the sidewalk. Stunned, I have to
be coaxed outside.

When John comes home late the next night, he walks into a charred
clearing where the garage was, where his car and bike and stored
photos of his family have gone up in smoke. I'm not there to meet
his summary loss because I'm holding Alek and desperately dreaming:
he's falling off a dock into a deep lake. I dive down after him, I won't
come up for breath. We're never found.

In the morning I ask Alek, "Did you dream?" He nods, head catching
halfway.

"A scary dream?"

Three more nods: his age. "I got under water."

"You did? How'd you get there?"

"I don't know," he says. "I came in in the middle."

It's for me to nod my stiff neck three times now. I understand that
a death, a fire, a dream of being saved from fire, then drowned, are
warnings of unforeseen consequences. Coming into the plot in the
middle, I seem to make the outcomes even worse. As *calor* and *rubor*
swell my nostrils and joints, I'm reminded that I refused to fly through
storms and thereby started a fire. That's the way it works, I whisper over
the charcoal of our ex-garage—the way it works with inflammation.
Inflammation signals the body to protect itself, stay home, lay aside
a hot bulb. But then it scorches everything by protecting it, leaving
burned-out ruins.

Immunity, 1985

I'm alarmed at how swiftly RA is consuming my joints. Osteoarthritis grinds down cartilage but doesn't inflame the whole neighborhood. Inflammation is what makes my disease so dangerous, and I've had enough flareups since Alek's birth that I now want to know what's bringing them on. If it's the action of overzealous immune cells, I should grasp why this shows up in weekly blood tests.

One week in the lab I say, as usual, "My name's here on the rand," pointing to a Rolodex file, when a strained voice behind me says, "Mine too." I turn to find a concave body in a wheelchair and know instantly what I'm seeing for the first time: a new disease. I'm seeing AIDS. I'm standing beside a young man with a name to be pulled off the rand.

As soon as they test each of us, I can't wait to go home, where I'm still living, where Alek is tumbling over the sofa with his best friend Manuel, five-year-olds on a tear. Falling into the ruckus, I remember AIDS stands for "acquired immune deficiency syndrome." I've heard how it's acquired, and I've just stood beside deficiency, and I can even grasp syndrome, but what I don't really get is immune.

"I better figure it out," I say.

"What?" shouts Alek.

"Why a pillow's flying at you," and I land one on his chest.

Everyone's saying "immune" in this new age of AIDS, but I have to know more, for it's a word that joins me to the young man I felt grief for in the lab. I read up, and late the next night say aloud, "Everything starts with antigens, with foreign particles that turn a body on."

John's eyebrows go up.

Antigens (I say, mostly to myself) turn on immune-system antibodies, the white blood cells at the source of inflammation. Usually antibodies keep security tight. When an antigen (the foreign particle) steps in, its surface (say, its backpack) has a suspect shape. A big immune antibody, or macrophage, processes the pack's contents, strews them around. This alerts the first-line patrol, helper T-cells, to grasp the antigen fragments by secreting helper-factor protein. Helper-factor recruits another squad, the B-cells, to fit themselves to the backpack, take notes on its shape, and store these in the permanent record. If the newcomer ever wanders in again, the B-cells nail it. Then a late shift comes on, immune-suppressor cells, to issue new orders—pipe down, drama's over—and the area returns to normal. Many times an hour, many times, the same scene recurs.

But my own immune system can't keep the lid on. In mine newcomers slip through patrols and use the space to reproduce. Or settled cells change shape and get attacked as strangers. Or patrols get excited and won't hold their fire. Or immune-suppressors aren't strong enough to shut them down. Or all of the above.

Then my thoughts turn back to the young man in my clinic's lab and his monstrous immune explosions. The new HIV epidemic knocks out the helper T-cells, leaving bodies immunodeficient, without their fight. In the strobe light of AIDS, RA's profile suddenly looks pretty sharp. Far from deficient, my teams of immune cells are so proficient they're overdoing the job. For the first time I'm impressed by that.

A week later, back at the lab for another gold shot, I glance around for the young man, then ask the overworked technician, "You've seen AIDS here?" meaning, "Is he alive?"

He answers, "They shouldn't act that way," and I know he means same-sex sex.

"Who shouldn't? Unknowing people? Newborns infected . . . ?"

"Newborns are innocent victims."

My God. What's a guilty victim? Presumably I too did something to deserve an immune disease.

On the way home from the lab I rave to myself in the driver's seat. Immune failures have brought centuries of wretchedness—leprosy in the thirteenth, plague in the fourteenth, syphilis in the sixteenth, TB in the nineteenth—but now, in the twentieth, AIDS has thrown us back ages, cursing the ill as sinners, damning homosexuals and addicts and prostitutes for spreading disease to the decent classes.

At home I walk through every peaceful place where I've hugged my family, until I land in my armchair and admit a frightening thought. We're bound together, this AIDS advent and my old news, this despised and migratory HIV and my stay-at-home RA. Both diseases bring forward aching joints as first signs. Both lose ground because of biased equations: AIDS = gay and arthritis = old. Both require urgent funds for research on immunity. Both derive meaning from the same conceptual jump, made some seventy years ago when Nobel laureate Paul Ehrlich foresaw autoimmunity. If the body confuses inborn with foreign, if it reads self as nonself, then the guardian immune system will decimate its host.

I cheer myself with one compensation: RA autoimmunities, as my doctor told me, are offering researchers a crucial edge on AIDS. Pulling myself from the armchair, I put Alek to sleep and blow a kiss into Sarah's room, then flop on our bed and say, "You know, John? I have a significant disease. I mean, RA is like an immune *efficiency* syndrome, which is why AIDS researchers want what RA's got."

"Let's see what RA's got right here," he says a minute later and coaxes my nightie off, rubs my shoulder, bends to kiss it, while my quickened desire knocks against pain. Later, grateful for a less deadly immune disease, I slip naked past the closet door with the full-length mirror inside. I'll just peep. Swollen ankle, thickening knees: check. Unmoving branch of wrist: check. What I'm seeing here—all the tussles among my cells, the helper, suppressor, and resident-alien ones— forms a model for our century's new maladies, the autoimmune kind, where bodies are trashed by their bodyguards.

The hardest lesson to learn from RA is that life-preserving forces ravage us, putting an end to endless possibility. "I have to learn this, but I don't have to look at it," I say and kick the closet shut.

Oddly enough, I do look at immunity, finally, in my own family sources, in the people I come from.

At a hundred-relative reunion in Cincinnati I ask an aging uncle if any relatives have disorders like mine. "Cancer everywhere," he says, "but nothing like that." I'm not relieved. Then he adds that we shouldn't grow older afraid of knowing who we are. "We're the outcome of your grandpa leaving Lithuania to seek happiness here."

"And did he find it?" I want to know.

"I have to tell you he glimpsed it and wrote his future father-in-law, 'Send your daughter. I got work teaching at Hebrew Union College.' The answer was *Never!* You get why?"

"Not really."

"Because his daughter was Orthodox Jewish. Hebrew Union College was Reform Jewish, like marrying outside the faith." My mind skips forward two generations, to the youngsters roistering past the corner where we're talking, happily tying the knot with any religion and gender and job lot. It's plain as a pie chart: my wider family's hardly Jewish anymore. That's the deregulating eighties for you.

"So what happened?" I ask.

"Your grandpa gave in and taught Orthodox school in Kentucky, on his feet all day. Your grandma arrived, and eight children later they were still kosher and penniless."

"But they got a place in America," I say. "Kids to be proud of." What if they'd stayed in Lithuania? Their story would have ended in 1941. No sequel here.

"El-eck!" someone calls, inviting my dad to talk with us about the old days. Back then, he tells us, teachers waved him away from college—too poor, too Jewish—and when he demanded, "What's the *best* place?" they said coldly: Yale. "Mary, I used all my savings getting there without knowing you have to be admitted. Then after fifteen entrance exams I paid by working in the infirmary and kept kosher by eating hard-boiled eggs."

"How long did *that* last?" A month?

"It's true the dean wanted to ban Jews, but what they really didn't tolerate was radicals."

And all at once I grasp the immunology term *intolerance*. Intolerant immune cells defend a body from outside incursion. But if they're *too* intolerant, like a biased college, they turn against clients they're supposed to serve. My dad's experience brings home the intolerant cells of RA, an illness I can't seem to grasp any other way.

Tolerant immune cells, on the other hand, resembling my later-generation family, want to live and let live. But if they're *too* tolerant, they let the system lose its core identity. They spell deficiency, like AIDS.

My dad goes on recounting the past: "You see, it was 1917, and I turned pacifist. That's what was tough as hell to be at Yale."

I lean against him because he needs thanking for his intrepid legacy. I could use it for owning up to RA, these days when what's tough as hell to be is immune-ill.

Shame, 1986

Brakes scream. A van I didn't see bears down on my car from the side, swerves wildly away. Given my stiff neck, I've steered into a parking lot without turning my head. I shudder from the near miss and slip unseen inside the supermarket.

At the checkout I'm behind two women lifting pint-size items with both hands. An express lane for arthritics? One shopper's fingers fumble a wallet and scatter change, a second one can't bend to pick it up, and a stiff-necked one escapes before anyone thinks she belongs here.

At home I call Ruth Rosen, my best friend, who always asks how I'm feeling as if she's taking a heavy platter out of my hands.

"How are you feeling?"

"Just now a van nearly smashed my car and—"

"Oh no. How?"

I mumble, "Neck—not so good." Knowing the answer's *always* arthritis stops me from owning up, as if it's a blot on my character. Among all the crooked features of my disease the one that still stands out is shame.

But why shame, if our checkout line's a common sight? A 1986 report in the *New York Times* informs me that handicaps hinder one in five Americans, from teenagers to senior citizens. The strange thing is, I'm the only person I know with my kind of handicap at my kind of age. So am I standard or oddball? I check a book on my shelf, Dr. Fries's *Arthritis: A Comprehensive Guide*, which assures me that arthritis brings "more work loss, more pain, and more poor functioning in daily life than does any other kind of human illness" and also that "more progress has been made in the fight against arthritis than in the struggle against all other major diseases." Huge claims, and news to me: I'm standard.

Then I toss a notebook in my book bag and head to Stanford Library. In twenty minutes I find a national ranking of "activity limitations," meaning chronic handicaps. Arthritis in all its varieties—osteo, rheumatoid, and others—is putting constraints on 13 percent of Americans in every age group, which I did not realize while driving under its influence. In a 1983 National Health Interview Survey arthritis easily comes out first and worst, for men or women, for incomes under ten thousand dollars but also for higher ones. It hangs heavier on Blacks but outweighs everything for everyone.

Pushing back my chair, I marvel at my belief that American joints stay in pretty good shape, except for mine and a few much older than mine. In fact RA commonly sets in from age twenty to age forty-five, and even osteoarthritis comes younger than we thought, often before forty-five, at least in women. It's a mystery, then, why I've kept mum about a top-ranking ailment for a good fifteen years.

One reason comes to me the next morning when I'm soaking my joints in a steamy bathtub and get stuck there. I bleat, "Someone?" and six-year-old Alek runs for John to slosh me out. Once on the bed I can't imagine a way to move off it. Spindly knees won't push me, sore arms can't hoist me, and there's nowhere to go from a roll. Hell, I whisper. No *word* can match this disease.

Somewhere in my nearby notebook I copied that idea from Virginia Woolf. "English which can explain the thoughts of Hamlet and the tragedy of Lear has no words for the shiver or the headache," she writes. "Language at once runs dry" or "will be something laughable." I tell the empty bedroom, "Aghhhh." All-the-time pain strains words of sense. In a poem I've copied out, Emily Dickinson writes, "Pain Has an Element of Blank."

Later, standing in the aisle of my local bookstore, I skim Elaine Scarry's 1985 book, The Body in Pain: "Physical pain does not simply resist language but actively destroys it, bringing about an immediate reversion to the state anterior to language, to the sounds and cries a human being makes before language is learned." Aghhhh . . .

I know chronic pain has trouble talking because I never reveal it to colleagues, scared they'll think I've carelessly permitted it to stay, worried they'll slip out of earshot. As Elaine Scarry writes, "To have pain is to have *certainty*; to hear about pain is to have *doubt*." It's unfair to let friends have doubt, or to bring kids home to the same gripes every afternoon. So I hold back. It shames me, having nothing good to tell, yet nothing bad enough.

What started me feeling this way, I think, was interviewing Holocaust survivors during two summers in Europe. While I was tracking the sealed cattle train that deported the painter Charlotte Salomon, I heard from an eyewitness that when it halted, the women were killed right away. So I learned for certain she lost her life in her first hour at Auschwitz. And I fainted. "Just recalling the Hitlerzeit," another eyewitness told me, "gives me pain. You understand? Pain." In the face of that agonizing "Hitler time" why would I ever mention my private creaks and groans?

"These are years of silence," I say to John one night. We're sharing spaghetti and parmesan, a no-slice no-chop dinner I can cook. These are years of silence, when I move from women's history to women's art to Charlotte Salomon to Nazism, and John switches from comic writers to Holocaust writers, and both of us come on pain so excessive it can't be voiced. At our cozy table we talk across Alek's head about anything but this.

"Your day OK?" is all I want to ask. We're sparing each other.

"Uh-huh." (He spends the day translating the Holocaust poems of Paul Celan.) "Yours?"

"OK." (I'm working through the Nuremberg trials, through Nazi language Celan called "the thousand darknesses of deathbringing speech.")

"How're your joints?" he asks.

"Not bad, not good." With practice muting news, I stay mum about this elbow on the table, bone to wood, missing its upholstery. I say, "Just show me you know." And he touches my knee, my shoulder.

The following morning I wake with forty million other Americans whose consciousness of day is consciousness of pain. I won't say anything, I tell myself. I'll feel better by afternoon. This afternoon we've planned an outing to the San Francisco Zoo, where it becomes clear how secretive I've been. I start snapping shots of Alek and a huge ox, while the beast keeps roaring and our peanut whining and

John insisting, "I must ask that musk ox." If he's the tongue twister
in the family, cheering us up, then I'm the album maker for the same
reason, happily clicking the point-and-shoot whose photos never catch
an image I don't want exposed, an image of my twisty hands or cocked
elbows. I hope to ban arthritis from every album in my household, from
everyone's memory, and from mine. So when Alek asks me to play wild
pouncing animals after the zoo, it's hard to confess, "I guess I don't
want to. It hurts my hands to pounce."

"OK."

"OK?"

"Let's play Lego." I'm so touched by his casual accepting of me-as-
I-am that I bleat, "Really?" He pats my hip. "You can go first."

Now Sarah's shouting from the front door, "Your mom and dad are
here!" Every night after dinner my parents walk to our house from a
rental in Palo Alto where I bring them to escape Pittsburgh's winter.
After hugging the grandchildren, they settle down for a long talk, the
kind we have nightly for two months every year, almost without the
word *arthritis*. Of course they're aware I have it, but I don't let on it
hurts.

I don't let on, to protect them. But the next afternoon, as I take a walk
with them, crunching my left foot to favor the right one, my mind runs
through the week's events, from the oncoming van to the unpictured
body and unvoiced pain. All of it (I now know) has conspired to put
me through weeks like this for fifteen years, with every act touched by
arthritis and still without breath to say the word aloud. For shame.

Shame leaves me formless and unarmed, feeling in my bones that
I'll be left behind.

I'd feel less shame if joints didn't come with jinxes. From the poet Ben Jonson: "May his joints tormented be." From *Hamlet* a curse that catches on: "The time is out of joint."

Aside from this, joints hardly rise into public view. Even their troubles settle near the ground like gravel, too low to keep an eye on. One reason, I'd guess, is that joints are hardly worth talking about, let alone whistling at. Like handles or gears they're the last thing we need a lot of slang for. And once they lose their spring, they drop contact with the power plant of sex. How can a person feel sexy when stiff in the shoulders and hips?

I bring this secret question home, where John's in the kitchen, frying up tofu for dinner. He looks good to me, better than the tofu. But how do I look? Frankly? Awful. It's been so many months, maybe years, since my body felt carefree that a sense of myself as exciting has dropped under the bed, mislaid. It's as if an inner eye needs to look me over and judge me desirable before I can feel desire for someone else.

As John puts out dinner (which Alek instantly abandons), I ask, "Sarah's still at her flute lesson?" John shrugs, and I count three nights this week he's showed up not quite knowing where anyone's been. Where's *he* been?

"John, I'm looking for sexy diseases, in novels or wherever."

"Sexy diseases? Gout?"

He's right. Gout was thought to keep company with gentlemen and claret.

"And consumption," John adds.

"Of what?" says Alek, and I laugh.

"Of lungs. It's an old word for tuberculosis." Yes, definitely consumption. Think of all those passionate heroines in operas—think of any with arthritis? Consumptives had such appeal that healthy women sometimes took arsenic to earn their flush, while consumptive men built up their bodies in the open air. If I've got it right, sex and exertion have always gained respect that no one ever won with creaky joints.

But I haven't got it right, because the neglect of arthritis is more than sexual—it's political. Social reformers hitched fast-moving TB germs to their causes, nothing less than the elimination of poverty, slums, filth. This could have been the case with rheumatic fever, an infectious form of arthritis that used to kill thousands every year. Often beginning with strep, rheumatic fever still strikes fifteen to twenty million people worldwide, mostly children from poorer places. But a divided world (chronic arthritis with public-health systems versus infectious arthritis without them) doesn't give any type much prestige.

The trouble with noninfectious arthritis is that it sticks to its own kind and keeps mum. When a disease is too aloof and stiff to inspire the body politic toward reform, I don't know why it would arouse any body at all.

After the tofu my parents arrive again. My dad settles on the couch beside me, his blue eyes and broad smile so like mine that John snaps a picture of us. I bless him for joking with my dad before heading to his office. But at the door beside him I can't help saying, "You run off every night to work while I stay here with my hands hardly writing anymore." Then I turn back inside. I'm losing my fluency—as a writer, as a woman. Stiff joints get in the way of both, of taking joy and inspiring someone else to.

Suddenly I need to know: why *am* I so stiff, anyway?

I pull my arthritis handbook from its bottom shelf and review what causes stiffness in rheumatic diseases. All parts of the joint get so inflamed they literally thicken up: my days start with "morning stiffness" (a polite phrase for cemented limbs), which breaks just in time for "afternoon gelling" (a sit-down that stays down). After months or years the stiffness settles in for good. That's why my toes winch up, elbows corner in, wrists tighten their turning circle.

Knowing this, I'm in awe of my mother as she teaches Alek a lotus pose, the same way she taught Sarah a decade ago. Perfecting yoga at age eighty-one, she's become a woman of spectacular litheness. In our living room she slides onto her back with one heel firmly on the rug, her other toe to the floor above her head. Then she spirals her torso around, pleased that she's gained the body of a gumband (as I was raised to call a rubber strip). Late in life her moving parts turn to pure elastic. Mine have given up their give.

But as she stretches like a feline in front of us, it's her mind that goes rigid, and I'm oddly grateful my stiffness stays in the joints. She keeps repeating questions to my dad, who happens to be hard of hearing.

"What's the time, dear?"

"How's that?" my dad asks.

"What time is it?"

"Huh? Eight o'clock."

"Oh yes. But the time, dear?"

"Huh?"

What a team. Then he tells me, "We all get older, Mary," nodding his head toward her. Suddenly she jumps up, stalks Alek here and there, haloing his head with her hands.

"Mom, why are you doing that?" I call out.

"Because he'll run into the doorknobs."

That does it. I decide to take her for an evaluation.

The next week a team of examining physicians pronounces a word she doesn't understand and my dad can't quite hear: "Alzheimer's." He shrugs and says, "We all get older, Mary." After that I also notice my mother's birch-tree body bulging at the tummy, but when she asks every few minutes, "Where's the bathroom?" I remember we all get older and let her be.

No one is listening to her anymore, I realize a few months later, when I get a frantic call from my dad in Pittsburgh. "A tumor's been growing, Mary." It's big as a honeydew now, pressing hard on her bladder. Where was her doctor all that time? For that matter, where was her daughter? Ashamed, I squeeze on a cross-country flight and speed to the hospital, where I face an odd tableau.

My mother is sitting up in bed—the tumor is benign—and asking why I'm here. Then she points fiercely to a Kleenex on the floor and hisses, "What's John Felstiner doing down there?"

What?

I need to get her out of the hospital before she's entirely nuts, and I do it that afternoon. That evening I put an arm under her shoulder and walk her step by step toward her kitchen, watching out for doorknobs. At one point she seems uncertain how to move, and my voice booms: "Try the right foot. Now your left. Right. Left." She comes to a dead stop where she stands, paralyzed, and takes no more steps, ever. I believe her last neural linkage blows out trying to translate my orders into motions for her legs.

A few days later I leave for home, leave my mother, all stiff like me, her suppleness gone the way of her wits. Turgor is starting to block my mind too, which at present won't bend around anything—like whether I can bear my mother's decline and if I missed John at our airport meeting place. Twenty minutes later he pulls up.

"Where the hell were you?" I shout.

"And how are you? Just fine?"

"Why can't you be on time?"

"I'm here, for chrissake."

I can't think what to say. It's his turn: "How did you leave your mother?"

"Oh John. In a wheelchair, confused. I have to go back."

Every night on the phone my dad cries for a wife whose brain no longer tells her legs to walk. And every night, yes, I blame myself—for commanding a left-right march (like ordering my own joints around) when all she needed to do was trust her gumband body one more time.

I cross the country again and again to see a person with no idea who I might be. So I apply myself to surveying the nursing home we've put her in. It looks like a rock sample of U.S. strata: invisible owners, for-profit managers, trained white nurses, African American aides, cleaners from another hemisphere, patients placed here thanks to working daughters and Medicaid. My dad tells the aides that his stiffened wife once hustled for civil rights, and I'm glad his pride keeps him boasting.

On the last day of my trip he takes his usual visitor's chair and reads snippets to her from the papers, as he always has. He asks me twice, "Isn't she beautiful, Mary?" as she babbles to her audience. It's not my dad or me—she never glances our way—but a little rag doll I brought for her.

"Mom, you want me to help you eat this spaghetti?"

Mom to doll: "Bye-bye."

"Bye-bye comes after lunch."

Mom to doll: "All in mary nix in."

"Nixon?"

To doll: "N-I-X-O-N."

"You can *spell* that? How come you still spell? Can you do . . . *spaghetti?*"

"S-P-A-G-H-E-T-T-I."

"I don't believe it."

To doll, sharply: "Bye-bye."

"Wait. Did you say *mary?* Mummy, you knew I was here."

"They've dragged her into Presby again," says my brother on the phone a month later, furious that the nursing home keeps sending her to Emergency. But I'm the one to rush to Pittsburgh and find her in Presbyterian Hospital, all skin and bones, stiff as steel, bed sores, too much for me. Then she's sent back to her "home," and I go back wearily to mine. A few weeks later we race through this routine again. One day, without a sign to anyone, she lets go.

What keeps coming back to me, for months after my mother's passing, is her pride in a flexible torso. Mine too looks light and easy and gives the impression I'm a pliant thing. Alone among my joints it bends without a snap. The legacy.

Distrust, 1987–88

To take my mother's matchless yoga body and vacuum her mind out of it—only a betraying Angel would pull that off. It's a sign that breaches of faith come in any form.

Even in my classroom I now suspect the worst. When I'm grading midterm tests and find two students misspelling "Bob Dylon," I figure one of them copied and send "See me" notes to both. Then a lesson in distrust begins.

Patricia is first to arrive: "Look, even my best friend copied off me."

"Linda's your best friend?"

"Yeah, and she's a cheater."

Later Linda sits in the same chair and says, "You *believed* her?"

"Well, shouldn't I?"

"No way. She copied me, accused me . . . then conned *you*."

I can't think what to say. Mistrusting my students, even these two, isn't the way the contract's supposed to work. I want to rely on them, on everyone. But after all my years blindsided by a disease I should know about distrust.

It's time to get on top of things like this. In a fever I commute home, buy groceries, cook dinner, call my dad, work with Sarah, tuck away Alek, sidle up to John—and let fly with all I've got. "WHY am I doing everything around here? Where are you all the time?"

"No place."

"John, just level with me."

"Too much work at the department."

"More than usual?"

"Well, yeah."

I let that pass.

The next day I meet with my student Patricia again. "It seems you copied your friend, then cut her loose"—she looks stunned—"so you need to talk to her in class."

But she stops coming to class. At semester's end a postcard from her says, "Professor. I have cancer now," which could be true or not. I send a long, kind letter (and sadly a failing grade). Then for months I keep mulling over her story, until I understand I'm dealing with my own set of disaffections. In my body the cells that guard me attack the joints that keep me moving. In my household the person who cared for my body edges away from it.

At night by long-distance I work at cheering my dad, who suffered a small stroke after losing my mom. I keep repeating, "You'll feel stronger."

"Not without her I won't." He's crying.

"Daddy, I promise, I'll take care of you." We go on this way for half an hour, always the same, every night.

I understand he's lost faith in his anatomy and feels alone in this distrust—the way I've been feeling for many months, out of connection with myself and John. Burrowing in his office, John won't spend free time with me, loses track of chores and family whereabouts. I can't rely on him anymore to be there for me or near me. These days he scarcely looks my way, seems all but moved out.

"Where *are* you?" I ask more than once.

"You just never lay off," he says, as if it's a moral flaw.

Am I the source of trouble after all? One way or another always out of joint?

At night I give John a light embrace, and though he responds, it's polite, inert. The moment I let go, he drifts away.

"John, what's going on?"

"I guess I'm tired."

"Tired? You run, swim, bike, hike."

"Mary, I don't know. I think I'm tired of—of your being less than you were. And you don't seem to want . . . well, sometimes I just want out."

"So where does this leave me? Married to an illness?" Damn it, I want out of RA too.

The next day, in sickness and in health (mine and his), I buy my first hardcover with "illness" in the title, Arthur Kleinman's new book, *The Illness Narratives*. I open it to find this: "The fidelity of our bodies is so basic that we never think of it—it is the certain grounds of our daily experience. Chronic illness is a betrayal of that fundamental trust. We feel under siege: untrusting, resentful of uncertainty, lost. Life becomes a working out of sentiments that follow closely from this corporeal betrayal: confusion, shock, anger, jealousy, despair." I copy this down because I know it's true. "Corporeal betrayal." My autoimmune physique, my stiffness, my uncertainty.

I feel seasoned in distrust, as if trained by my disease. Warily I watch our old contract fading, John counting himself out and then shutting me out. For months Alek notes us sharing a room but hardly a word. Sarah arrives for vacation and hears an empty assurance: "It'll be OK."

I know all long relationships fray as a matter of course, and the extra strain of illness can snap them in two.

But I want my joints to bind ours all the closer. If we give up, it's like saying the strains are my fault. If we let a marriage founder on innocent illness, we split a family that's taken us through thick and thin. At the very least I need a cohesive household for my daughter in college, my first-grade son. And I'd choose the same for myself too, since my heart hates to be abandoned and so do my joints. Yet I can't settle only for that. There has to be love moving between us, hand to hand.

Finally John agrees to couples therapy, a miserable experience for both of us. What he hates is feeling in the wrong. What I hate is moral balancing, as in, "That's one way to see it, Mary. And how do you see it, John?" After many sessions like this we arrive at make-or-break:

> John: "It seems I'm the one who has to do the changing."
> Therapist: "And how do you see it, Mary?"
> Mary: "He's the one who has to do the changing." I hold my breath.
> John: "Then what's *Mary* have to do?"
> Therapist: "Mary has to decide whether she wants to be with you."
> Mary (to herself): Thank you thank you. Finally.

Months of quiet indignation, and not so quiet, go by without our getting to the bottom of what's happened. Alone I pace the hilltop near our house, muttering to myself. Is he sick of being close to someone sick? How could he turn against my body when my body's turning against me?

One morning I wake to see John looking my way. "How are you?" he whispers. "Are you hurting?"

"Both shoulders." I can't manage to share details with someone who's spent nearly a year looking away. But his eyes fill with so much pain I'm pierced by his empathy—not because it keeps me going, though it does, but because it's part of him and I love that. I realize I couldn't bear to *watch* arthritis as he does.

"Mary, I want to tell you this. Avoiding you, in a way, it's avoiding turning fifty. And I must be escaping the abrasion—the daily—the abrasion of your disease."

"Well, I don't get to do that." I move away from him. I don't like his fear of decline in himself and in me, or his warding off frailties by going it alone.

"Your shoulders?" he asks and reaches out to massage.

"Never mind." I roll to the edge of the bed. I do want this bond to last, but I can't stop my outraged heart from stiffening like my hands.

After many more talks like this I reach a kind of judgment. Against John for retreat and cover-up when he had all his health. Against myself for losing touch with him when physical ease deserted me, for taking out on him my endemic fury and shame. Against John for letting my illness sap his faith, turn him away. Against myself for begrudging his liberty, for cranking my needs into orders. Against John for weakness verging on defection.

So when a former student phones to complain she now has arthritis, I'm not surprised by her very first thought: "Who would want to live with me?" Precisely. Women with handicaps, she reminds me, are less likely—oh much less—to feel wanted; they're likelier to divorce and lose child custody. Once divorced, she tells me, women with RA remarry less than other women.

I never lose sight of this or of the strains that chronic illness places on partners, yet slowly, slowly, love does seep back in. If now is the worst we go through, we *have* come through.

One afternoon on a walk in the hills my friend Margo shouts over the rustling trees, "The important thing is, Mary, you're resilient."

"Brazilian?" I shout back. A strong wind blows "Girl from Ipanema" through my mind, and my faulty feet break into a samba.

Morbidity, 1988

Day by day John and I keep fixing our friendship and (in the same makeover spirit) fixing a cabin in the Santa Cruz Mountains, an hour from home. After awhile, when we're used to joking again and tumbling into bed, I invite my dad to visit.

He arrives looking so bereft I take him outside and ask on impulse if he wants to say *Kaddish* for my mother. Scanning the forested ridges, this old atheist holds my hand and runs flawlessly through the Hebrew prayer for the dead. Then he thanks me, and we break out some hot dogs. Because it's the Fourth of July and Reagan's vice president wants to climb the job ladder, my dad regains his spitfire. We celebrate resistance in a loud reading of the Declaration of Independence, then the 1848 Seneca Falls declaration of women's rights, whose great insight still hits home: pain that women suffer privately is also systemic.

Even pain in our bodies, I'm thinking, gets worse with prejudice. I've heard people label certain ailments trivial or mythical, calling chronic fatigue syndrome a lot of women acting tired or writing off fibromyalgia as a fancy name for depression.

I also tell my dad that only 13 percent of government research funds go to mainly female illnesses.

He looks impressed. "How did you learn that, Mary?"

"I'm a teacher, Daddy, I take notes." Actually I'm not sure why I copy out percentages, since I don't teach women's health or write about it. What I do is scribble bits and pieces on scraps. I take down the fact that we test drugs on male-only subjects, then prescribe the pills to women. I note we make men the measure, labeling their hearts heart-sized, women's hearts smaller, and we use catheters to save ten men's hearts for each woman's. As I watch my dad tuck into a no-nitrite hot dog, I remember that women, the bulk of the poor, grow ill with bad food and high stress. I've noted the wretched skewing of healthcare that lets white women live six years longer than African American ones.

Ah, I see what I've been doing: I've been building a prosecution case. "When women get chronically ill, officials hardly cock an ear."

"It's bias?" my dad asks, baffled.

"It's bias when making do with, say, achy arthritic joints is *expected* of us, like managing the kids or putting up with—uninterested men."

John steps back. "Don't women outlive us?"

"Not always," my dad says softly.

"Oh Daddy. Those extra years women live are most often sickly ones."

He shakes his head. "Taken too soon, your mom."

But I'm thinking: she was spared.

"My dad visited with us and said *Kaddish*," I tell my friend Ruth on her answering machine across the bay. "Let's talk." Our habit is to dial each other every week and hear a little wit, a little coziness. Whenever gloom gets the better of me, Ruth calls to say, "Just be proud of Alek in second grade and Sarah in her second year at Yale." These days, with my mother gone, my father weepy, the love of my life iffy, the daughter of my heart far away, Ruth coaxes me out of being morbid, if that's what I am. *Morbid* from *morbidus*, which in twelfth-grade Latin meant "diseased." I think I own the word.

One night I pick up the receiver and hear a whisper: "Mary."

"Ruth? What's going on?"

Two words: "Breast cancer." She doesn't dare say them again.

I jackknife out of my seat. Then, trying to sound reassuring, I tell her how many other friends with breast cancer have solidly recovered.

After the call panic spills. I pump through my empty rooms yelling, "You will not take her away. You drop illness on *me*. Understand?" These words collapse to "Angel, I beg you. Please."

In the next months my best friend burns through chemotherapy, and I feel the Fahrenheit rise in my joints. As radiation bullies her body, my body doubles up. She's the one threatened, I'm the one in pain. I'm the lucky one. After a long while it dawns on me she isn't marching to the scaffold that very hour. Chemicals are poisoning her cells so they'll recover. Morbid is what this moment is, I tell myself, not mortal.

A few months later I seem to be of two minds—feeling bonded to Ruth but wanting to spring away—and of two bodies too. One of them strides the khaki hills, its lightness rising from methotrexate, a new medicine to replace gold and sprinkle on top of antimalarials. But my other body, the one that feels radiated along with Ruth, waits in the wings and mistrusts this summer flush. It knows new medications lose their fizz.

On a warm weekend when John says, "Let's hike," my first body flies out to him, and we tramp over footpaths and cowpaths, my legs going all-terrain. Then a skip to the road lands on my left ankle, which buckles instantly. John carries me to the car and to the clinic, where my foot's sealed in a cast. But it's just a hike, a leap, a break, and nothing to do with disease.

Later my rheumatologist puts another twist on it. "It fractured when your joint refused to flex. And because your bones are thinned by RA."

"Oh no. I was feeling so . . . I don't know . . . off the leash!"

"Well, now you need to think about replacement hormones."

"No, I don't," I shoot back. "I'm barely starting menopause." At my first missed periods I suspected pregnancy, not the start of the end of maternity. Now I'm joining thirty million so-called menoboomers, though the ones I know don't live with thinning bones, whereas I can alphabetize the friends with breast cancer. Which I feel wide open to. And taking hormones raises the risk.

Dr. B. says, "Taking hormones will slow osteoporosis, which runs with RA."

It runs with RA? Is my free pick either crumbling bones or cancer risk? I turn stubborn. "Since I had flareups after pregnancy, shouldn't menopause damp it down?"

He shakes his head. "Arthritis hits women hardest when they're oldest."

What hits me hardest is the shock to my best friend, more than to myself. Even refusing hormones reacts first to the illness that's hers.

Gently my doctor peels off the ankle cast, and almost at once a painful swelling arrives to take its place. Within weeks it spreads to the point where it can't be trimmed back: from the ankle it bubbles up the leg, then jumps from knee to hip to shoulder. As I limp painfully down the block, hardly believing I climbed hills a few weeks ago, a hard question knocks at me. Is my RA recharged by a sprain, or by menopause, or is my problem mental stress? In the last years I've faced distrust in my household, pushed women's history through doubting committees, grown sick on the Holocaust, endured a fire, buried a mother, carried a father, feared for a friend, and in the thick of this, well, the joints held on. Only *afterward* they're getting testy. I hear that rats with collagen arthritis (the ratty form of RA) actually grow stronger when exposed to felines. What makes the poor things sick, though, is constant noise. Maybe for me a loss of quiet in the air—a cumulative want of trust—has opened the system to full disease.

I'd like to know how lack of trust transmits itself to joints (no one is describing this). For me it probably begins at night, with general fear startling me awake until my mind finds reasons for anxiety (personal and political) and keeps disrupting sleep, so that I begin the day too tired for exercise, which leads to weakness that makes for fear of losing control. Caught in this cycle, my RA lives up to its nickname: the Crippler. What distinguishes the Crippler is its assembly of musculoskeletal *and* rheumatic features; it combines the mechanical breakdowns of osteoarthritis with the unpredictable flarings of autoimmune disease. Where all forms of arthritis make for misery, where osteoarthritis wears away cartilage around specific joints, where gout makes crystals in the spaces between them, where psoriatic arthritis hardens the skin and joints, where ankylosing spondylitis inflames the spine and sometimes fuses the bones, where lupus attacks internal organs, where fibromyalgia squeezes the neck and surroundings, here's the Crippler, still out front, swelling the synovial membranes, vexing the joints underneath, then going for cartilage, ligaments, and tendons. Then the ends of bones.

It's a good thing only two million arthritis sufferers in this country have the Crippler, for they're the ones who go into swift decline. Doctors try new drugs that soon lose oomph. Patients ask, How much worse can it get? Doctors say, Much worse. Patients think, At least not *cancer*. Doctors think, Actually, this too invades the tissue and destroys it.

"Morbidity," I tell my dad on a visit to Pittsburgh, "is the word I've learned for both sickness and sorrow, like *dolor* for pain and for grief . . ." I stop quickly and survey the city from my dad's little terrace, the rustbelt of steelworks fallen to disuse and two, maybe three hospitals at any glance. Even the begonias in his planters look limp and unemployed.

"I have to water them all the time," my dad says, holding the hose too long over each flowerpot.

"They have a great view here."

"But I'm moving out there with you, Mary." Just like that.

"No, you're not." Just like *that*. I can't imagine my household with one needy dad, two shortchanged kids, many painful joints. My answer shoots from the hipbone.

"Whatever you want, Eleck," John adds gently.

"I'll think on it," he says as if he has years and years to think. "Mary, I'll make some wieners for your lunch, Mary."

The next morning Ann breezes in, a vibrant woman hired after my dad's recent stroke, when he joined nine million Americans who can't make it on their own. He's lucky to have her around. She's asking, "Eleck, what's the score?" and she means this. Ann has him watching sports, shoulder to shoulder on the sofa, and he has her pinned to news, a new trick for each of them. When she goes home for weekends, he goes too. "At your place," she teases him, "I cook low-fat, and at *mine* you eat pork fat." Soon he's a fixture among her inner-city friends, who buzz his phone all week: "Eleck, my man!"

How does my eighty-nine-year-old dad welcome new foods, new teams, new neighborhoods, when at forty-eight I'm already stiff and cautious?

I ask him before I leave Pittsburgh, "How do you do it?"

"Always fight back."

Against what? I can't cure my disease, at its lowest point in twenty years of morbidity. How do I know what to fight against?

Mortality, 1989

This is more or less what I'm asking at Yom Kippur, the last Day of Atonement before the 1980s go away. "All rise," calls the rabbi, and about fifteen hundred people in a Stanford auditorium rise to atone. I sit cold as an apostate: Not me, Lord, unless new knees are provided here. Then a brief flash comes down, maybe from the Angel of Anatomy. Might the universe *need* my creaky, self-destroying joints? At least they tend not to break into others' lands and can't do harm to the environment. They could be sustaining the ecosystem. Yes, lowly ligatures make good models. Hang together, they urge. Only connect.

I have to admit it's the first time they've shone in this light. So if I've cursed them a wee bit in the past, I think I've just atoned.

After Yom Kippur I start teaching my first course on genocide, hoping to soften some flinty students by asking how, in their opinion, humans resist destroying each other.

"Like fish!" shouts one of them. "Make themselves hard to catch."

Everyone waits for me to respond. "Well, OK, but one difference . . ." I try. "Humans attribute meaning to destruction. *Fish don't.* Think if your own existence was menaced." No one speaks.

The student stares out the window, repaying my "Fish don't."

A scowling, head-shaven classmate lifts a finger to his throat and slits.

Two women in the front show me they're making notes, not taking notes.

The teacher starts wondering if only students can drop a class.

Last shot: talk about Charlotte Salomon under the Nazis. "When she knew she might die, she invented an audience to show her life to, a mythical *You*."

At the end of class a kindly student leans close and whispers, "*You* are her *You*."

Does that mean if I could find a You I might do the same sort of job, narrating my private pain? My mind swiftly puts the idea aside. Of course joint pain can't compare with the suffering of Nazi victims. Mine's internal, theirs was inflicted. Mine won't lead to death. Theirs did.

But even as I make these distinctions, the genocide course keeps blurring them. One day a Jewish student confides that reading Nazi propaganda makes him feel "unfit and ugly." He says, "I can't imagine why my girlfriend sticks around."

"Could you maybe check with her?"

He does, and her answer ("We all should be so ugly") appears to hearten him, but he still fears visceral disgust toward "certain faces, certain builds."

I think silently, No one envies my bent-up joints or my nice slow way of moving them.

After awhile he asks, "What did Nazis kill sick people for?"

"They thought the sick and disabled"—a group that must have included some arthritics—"were almost like Jews: life unworthy of life." Suddenly the words *Jewish* and *sickish* snap together in me, along with *unfit*, *ugly*, and *unworthy*.

"What made Nazis call others unworthy of living?" I ask the silent genocide class, missing the warmth of my other students, and then I raise the question differently: What created SS killers?

A camouflage-clad student answers fast: "Officer tells you to kill, you kill." In a split second he cocks an index finger near a female student's neck.

"Get offa me, you freak."

"Yeah. And if I was SS, I'd do everything they told me to."

In shock, all I come up with is, "No threats allowed here. We have to move on." Right now what I need is a hall pass. No, a sick leave, the excuse at least of arthritis.

Retreating to my office, I find things getting worse. During class an expensive transcriber, used for my dictation tapes, has vanished from my desk, leaving me alienated from my means of production. "Lifted," I tell the campus policeman who comes around. "It's a disaster for someone who can't use her hands." He makes a note, then stretches out to talk.

"So this isn't a busy day?" I ask. It is for me.

"Boring. Not a blip." He takes off.

Four hours later I hear a rustling on all sides. A pile of midterms (uncorrected) slips off the shelf. A sudden slanting sends me to the doorjamb, bracing for safety. Megaphones blare, "Earthquake! Go!" and I speed outside. Somewhere out here my police officer is handling this blip.

On the freeway I listen to sickening news of commuters crushed by roads and bridges. Alek—my God, is he safe? John? Speeding home, I see the quake has struck close. Inside the house mirrors are shattered, vases spilled, shelves skeletal, and John stock-still, whispering, "The force of it."

"Alek? Where?"

"Upstairs. I brought him from school. At home, just sitting here, I slammed the wall." That's four feet from his desk. His body is hurt. So is this house.

How badly hurt becomes clear the next day with the yellow tape. "We're looking at condemning the whole structure," says a police officer. Then an insurance adjuster arrives. "Do I know you . . . Felstiner?" he asks abruptly at the door.

"Me and John?"

"Right! Right! I served under Lieutenant John in the Navy. So Mrs. John, let's see what needs fixing here." I gasp. It's a remission.

What we need is ground-up retrofitting, and the adjuster approves full payment (his salute). The frame will be jacked in the air for half a year, the foundation hacked away, the house inched down on a new base, and the residents told to resume their lives.

But tectonic grinding has set the joists off angle, and under the foundation runs a continental fault. At any time—I know this now—we can be condemned.

A few days later, when my genocide class meets again, aftershocks that could be earthquakes roll under our seats. We need to make a collective exit plan, but we're at odds. My camouflage-clad student hisses, "Whatever half-assed plan you make, I want outta here." The whole quarrelsome group looks my way, and a terrible knowing sparks their eyes. Tossed together in disaster, threatened by a monstrous force beyond control, suddenly we touch what has escaped us all along: a sense of genocide.

My face, my bones, feel crushed. Making my way slowly to the office, I'm not surprised to see Camouflage waiting: "What I said in class—"

"What you said in class was bullshit. You'd be the last to leave." Now I *am* surprised: he's crying.

"How'd you know that?" he says. I shrug. I know because my useless arms and legs will want to protect my students, and my mind picks him to do the job.

"And about obeying the SS?" he goes on. "If they forced me at gunpoint to kill, I'd kill *them*."

"I believe you would. So now you know how you'd act under threat to life. It's momentous, finding out."

Then I'm the one who has to find out, from another sort of after-shock. Another of the students, the head-shaven one, spikes his last assignment with swastikas, labels the multiethnic group "your nigger and Jew class," names "you, Jew" as the kind of person he's "wanting to kill."

I rush to the department chair, who suggests I dress the student down. But another colleague makes fussy noises about free speech, while yet another looks me straight in the eye and says I should *not* assign free writing. On my own I ask mental-health counselors: Could I help the student? The counselors tell me, No contact: he'll think you're weak and attack.

I hold up crooked little hands: I *am* weak.

Then I decide to demand his expulsion. The disciplinary officer says: Good plan, except he's probably packing a pistol. So I ask the arm of the law for protection. The police mention they cannot protect me.

I take my sorry joints down the hall and admit I'm defenseless. I'm RA-minded: weak-kneed.

After all the careful distinctions in my course, terms like *helpless* and *victim* are leaking onto me. I take myself home, look over the student's earlier work, decide it's not all bad. If this is a moral test, I spend it thinking my nine-year-old shouldn't lose a mother to a teacher's principle. Forget the skinhead's viciousness. Forget the always-fight-back ideal. Forget everyone's duty to resist Nazis from the first day. Give the guy a B.

So now I know how to act under threat to life. Just cave in.

Not a word of this passes to my dad when he calls from Pittsburgh, because every night he's crying. "Mary, I miss your mom. I miss *you*."

"I know, Daddy." Pause. "How's Ann? How's sports?"

One night after one of these talks he settles in his armchair while Ann trims his hair, and as he turns KDKA extra loud for his hourly news, his heart fails. There's no pain in his final moments, and Angel, I give thanks for that.

Over the next weeks I keep recalling his fight-back words and how he lived them and how I don't. My spirit seems wafer thin: it follows my body into a habit of feeling weak. While arranging a memorial service in Pittsburgh, I also discover my fragileness has some roots. As I clear my parents' apartment with my brother, I come on an ancient "Dear Mary" from him, railing at me as a child for not always taking his side. This note strikes me as a source text for my lifelong terror of bullies, up to a recent skinhead.

After my brother leaves, for two more weeks I live with my parents' belongings, trying to catch my dad's voice: "Mary, I'll make wieners for your lunch, Mary." Bereft, I ship home a dresser with a hundred pairs of my mother's hosiery and then slowly empty the closets. I'm getting to know my family too late, sifting through notes from long-gone lectures (a lifetime service record), coupons from Giant Eagle (five cents off canned grapes), RSVPs from my wedding twenty-three years ago, decades of monthly prepaid rent receipts. Clearing my parents' holdings, I suddenly see they've left me a testament called You Never Know.

At that moment I vow to ditch my own detritus before my children have to do it: my disused sporting goods, my archive of past prescriptions, my armory of old insurance forms, my tight-fitting pre-RA clothes. I plan to thrust my hands into drawers and files, plump the garbage bags, sink the recycling center. A friend asks, astonished, "You'll give away things you might need again?"

"The fact is, I won't," because mine's a body that isn't going to change for the better. And because for the first time I know the ball bounces and I'll pass on.

Back at home my first move is to weed out all the expired prescription bottles, so I'll be ready when my body says, Past this date, dispose. There's no reason to worry quite yet: my family longevity looks pretty good. My grandparents survived to old age, succumbing to heart failure and cancer. My mother made it all the way into Alzheimer's. Between those generations and mine came a great demographic shift, doubling my shelf life. And of course my carefulness should work against the major threats, like HIV, alcohol, suicide. I'll be good.

That's when I find out I can't be good enough.

In the basement of Stanford Medical Library I take a peek at mortality figures, hoping a medical textbook will confirm my chance at long life, like my parents. But instead I find 1989 studies of RA chewing up that chance. Rarely do RA patients recover, and most decline into disability after just five years. What's worse, no one notices their early expiration date. RA is an indirect cause that isn't listed on death certificates. So patients and politicians don't realize arthritis kills.

It kills.

With RA the blood-vessel linings swell, causing heart attacks. Cancer occurs two to three times more often, and mortality is even higher for women than for men. Compared to healthy people, those with severe RA die younger by ten to fifteen years. The Angel has it in for us.

I come home with these figures and stand outside the door of my house, ignoring "Mom?" and "Mary?" Then I step off toward the hills. Among the darkened greens of late winter I'm forced to see life menaced—my best friend's cancer, my parents' deaths, a skinhead's threat, the earth shaken like a backbone. Having RA, I thought, was my personal shield against You Never Know, my prepaid rent receipt. Yes, it brought home morbidity, but my ailing parents kept me a generation away from mortality.

When they were alive, I had a disease. Now it has me. Now I'll be infirm, in pain, in want of fifteen years it'll take away. Morbid falls much nearer to mortal than I used to think. An Indo-European root word may link the two, and only sheer hope keeps them separate.

So what can I do? I've already put my mind to inflammation and immunity, put my finger on shame, gotten wise to silence and pain, to the exponential power of distrust, to the shortening of my days. And I still live right on a fault. What can I do except brace in doorjambs, give out Bs, cover my ears against the cosmic wingbeat coming to pick me off?

III. Getting Back

Oh, there were tricks in every trade,
more than one way ...
to outwit rheumatoid arthritis.

Henry Roth,
Mercy of a Rude Stream

Access, 1993

It takes a new decade before my mind finally warms to my father's idea of fighting back. First I remember poet Audre Lorde: "Battling racism and battling heterosexism and battling apartheid have the same urgency inside me as battling cancer." Then there's Susan Sontag's new book on AIDS, which speaks of battling the fear of diseases "regarded as deviant." What I seem to be doing is gathering intelligence for a skirmish, building a little arsenal of knowledge. It dawns on me I could fight back, against a complex enemy. It's personal: it's called shame. It's political: it's called neglect.

And with that realization an intricate struggle begins.

In my office I say to Julio, a typist cofinanced by me and my school, "Maybe I ought to push the state for more help. I guess I need the new law on my side," meaning the Americans with Disabilities Act, passed in 1990 after wheelchair protests and political push. A brochure I read to Julio shows the ADA mandating "reasonable accommodation" for any employee with "a physical or mental impairment that substantially limits one or more of the major life activities."

"That means . . . what?" Julio asks.

"That means my employer, within reason, has to make my job of writing and teaching accessible to me."

"So you want me to type a request?"

"Go ahead, fire up the computer. Let's ask my boss to provide me reasonable accommodation, in the form of a typist with more hours and pay. Here goes."

> Dear State of California:
> As I'm unable to use my hands for writing or typing, owing
> to severe rheumatoid arthritis, I need a clerical assistant
> during my upcoming sabbatical. . . .

OK, Julio, cross your fingers—another trick his fingers do for mine. But
he prefers a karate kick and a grunted warning: "Send her the money."

In the next weeks I find out which illnesses count for the ADA. So
far, cases of diabetes, breast cancer, and epilepsy have all fallen short
in the lower courts. And arthritis? An answer arrives when I'm in my
office again with Julio.

Request for Reasonable Accommodation: Denied.

"Bitch," says my typist.

"We could look at it from their point of view," I say.

"Their point of view is no."

"The thing is, this new law follows the '64 Civil Rights Act but takes
actual money to comply with—ramps, wheelchair lifts, karate typists—
so the state narrows its scope, excludes a sabbatical. The irony is I'm
researching interwar Germany, which by the way set hiring quotas to
support the disabled."

"Sounds good."

"Until the Third Reich excluded my race and sex."

"Not so good."

"The ADA calls for access, not quotas, and that suits me fine. I'll just
send an appeal to remind California: You goofed."

"Go for it. Dictate."

> Appeal:
> In denying me clerical assistance during sabbatical, the
> State denies me the use of sabbatical. This is unjust.

Arriving home later, I believe I've nailed the ADA's point. Disability
turns into discrimination if my employer refuses to clear the way for my
functioning. As I throw myself into the overstuffed armchair, a question
I've avoided catches me. Am I disabled? Probably not. Probably my
state won't help me because my nontyping hands just drove me home.
Disability isn't my issue anyway. Mine's disease. So I shrug and wait for
administrative mills to stonegrind a solution.

Reasonable Accommodation Appeal: Denied.

I give up. I pay my typist out-of-pocket, overuse my hands, learn
to be reasonable and accommodate. And somehow during 1993, by
dictating every word, retaping to revise, checking typescripts, taping
again, in a process too slow to stand, I finish a biography of Charlotte

Salomon, whose life and death knock to pieces any self-pity I might be leaning on.

One day I peek into *No Pity*, Joseph Shapiro's lively 1993 book, which quotes a disability activist: "Playing to pity . . . raises walls of fear between the public and us." Of course I imagine I'm the public and not "us." Then I find out my department has hired Paul Longmore, a historian who can't use his arms because of polio, who publicly burned his own book to protest the state cutting his benefits when he earned royalties. "A disability activist is coming to where I work," I tell John.

"You're in for some changes," John says.

Paul Longmore's voice fills the history department office when I first hear it. I whirl around, and my mind trips over itself. If he's disabled, then I'm not: I'm straighter, taller, handier, and I open my own mail. My body just a has a few little wrongs.

His body, I notice, has rights. I see his unabashed look and want to know where he got it from.

After we've made friends, he recounts how disabled students and teachers couldn't reach their classes until they started demanding access in 1970s Berkeley. While I was busy hiding my handicap, he didn't have that choice. Someone once told him, "If I were you, I'd kill myself," which I guess he thought was bad advice.

I ask him for better advice, since I've been wanting to know: how does he handle writing without the use of his hands?

"I lie on the bed," he says, "with a pen in my mouth and a ventilator for my lungs."

Suddenly my maddening tape recorder seems a cinch. "I'm lucky, I guess. Whatever I want to do I still do—except write, type, cook." Paul smiles at these things I shouldn't be deprived of and says that a body's problems need solutions, namely access. But I insist, "This is an *illness* limiting me, not a barrier."

"Some of each," he says.

"I've just heard," I admit, "that RA patients can't get disability payments. One out of two is turned down. I mean, we're expected to take pain today and damage tomorrow and get on with the job. And half the people with RA lose a good part of their income, like me." I'm thinking of how many semesters I've had to cut back courses and salary. He shakes his head, and I get it: a disease alone couldn't make *half* of us poorer. A failure of fairness does that.

Just knowing someone who openly demands access for a disjointed body—well, that starts changing my life. We move slowly into a department meeting together. I cock my T-square elbows on the table for everyone to see, and for the first time I'm not all that ashamed.

A few days later I call my friend Ruth: "Do you realize we live at the core of a militant disability movement?" Ruth does realize, knowing of Berkeley's Center for Independent Living. Then I call a colleague who can tell me about it, because "independent living" sounds impossible to me. My colleague says the center is run by residents, "like Het Dorp in Holland, which also welcomes chronic diseases."

I tell her quickly I have one of those. Then I can't help asking, "Do they live there on their own?"

"California funds attendants, the first state to do it."

"That's great," I say. "At home it's my partner making things work."

"You know, you have a right to get outside help."

A right? Wounded veterans have a right, maimed workers. Everyone else depends on the kindness of . . .

"You have a right," she says.

But I'd like this right without admitting physical faults. A little contradiction there?

Finally I compose a mental lesson called, Why Support the Impaired? It goes like this: We can't abolish impairments, and we need the unfittest to broaden human variance (time to turn Darwin on his head), because the more the spectrum stretches, the more normal every one of us will look. Then it strikes me that the prime question in these times—who gets equal opportunity?—is moving toward a brand-new solution. Rights must go out to every body, to senior bodies and kids' bodies, to queer and straight ones, to the hued and the pale faced, the lame and the buff. And that means to me.

By now my old safeguard—nobody knows my trouble—seems to have lost its use. There's no point pretending I can pass, all handicaps hidden, when I'm on the examining table of a consulting rheumatologist. He speaks two words that throw me back twenty-four years, to the first time RA stunned me into silence.

What he says is, "The wrists."

Despair, 1993

"What *about* the wrists?" Their slimness holds my gaze.

The famous rheumatologist says, "They're eroded. They're narrow." Not slim but narrow, a world of difference. My admiration slips off the examining table to be swept up by a janitor.

"Your x-rays show worn-down cartilage, bone, and muscle mass. I'd strongly recommend prednisone."

"Cortisone! But it's dangerous . . . OK." Remarkable how fast a shocked patient accedes: I suddenly see my real arms, skinny at the wrist and pulpy at the elbow, a grandmother's arms at a mother's age, classifying me as someone who'd better not wait around. I'm told these nineties rheumatologists go for kick-butt treatments. Crush the disease before it makes inroads, crush it after, send in the steroids. Right on this table I'm seeing a startling reversal of the treatment pyramid, unchallenged since the sixties, when I started inching up it. No longer is joint destruction considered a wiser course than dangerous drugs. Even harmless aspirin, this physician explains, turns out to be much less safe than people thought, while a strong drug like methotrexate turns out safer. Aspirin unsafe? But I don't want to know. It seems I can't get by with what I've done before. I must try cortisone to strengthen my wrists—and then think of something to muscle up my spirit.

I start with a simple dare: take a nice look at listed side effects. Well, well, while deflating the synovial lining of joints, cortisone can puff up faces, rouse hunger, weaken muscles, soften bones, invite ulcers. So far in me it merely creates midnight panics where the heart scuds, the feet jerk, the sleeper wants to bolt. I seem to have topped off the treatment pyramid, moving from a dozen-odd aspirin to antimalarials, through gold and methotrexate, to a heavy-duty steroid. If this doesn't work, I think there's nowhere higher to go.

A few months later I'm in the air above the ocean, flying with John and Alek to spend spring at Stanford's campus in England. Taking a window seat, I'm looking for dizzier views, hoping to become wiser because of them. I want inspiring sights in England, like the arthritis-openness of Bath twelve years ago. Because visions rarely arrive by way of arthritis, I'm happy to be taken by surprise.

Our first morning in the venerable marsh called Oxford, we pass a neighbor digging around her icy flower beds. In my black parka, wool scarf, and two sweaters—this is April—I warm my jaws by calling to her, "How are the daffodils?"

"They've all gone over," she says, shaking her head.

"To the other side?" John asks mournfully, as a spectral bus comes through the fog to take us to the library. In a cold booth I'm snapped for an ID photo that shows my smile stopped by broad cheeks. To my eye the camera pierces reality: this sad, fat face is all my fault. Staring at my lumpy, downcast self, I think I'm unpardonable.

The next day, when our daffodil neighbor asks, "Are you churchgoers?" as casually as asking if we're sports fans, I rush to answer, "I'll go." It might help twelve-year-old Alek in school, where chapel starts the days, where non-Christians wait in an anteroom, a little closet.

"You alone there?" I ask.

"There's a Muslim boy."

"And what are you two missing besides hymns?"

"School announcements. You might as well be Christian here," he tells me.

During Easter services in a stone-cold church I might as well be Christian too and bless my troubles. Blessed be the ankle, I whisper, the elbow, the knee. But they stay too stiff to move, and I feel cursed by growing colder, along with the spring.

One chill morning, to clear the curse, I go looking in a science library, where I wind toward the shelves and stop in my tracks. I can't lift down the medical books to find out why I can't lift down the medical books. Among the silent researchers I hear a whimper coming from my place.

With every joint aching, my fingers actually feel *The Problem of Pain*, by C. S. Lewis, which many readers before me have found inspiring enough to underline. "What is good in any painful experience for the sufferer, is submission to the will of God, and for the spectators, the compassion aroused and the act of mercy to which it leads." Uh-oh. A submission-compassion model would hold me down so others can learn charity. Pulling my parka close (it's late May now), I'm forced to ask: What is "good in any painful experience for the sufferer"? An answer steps right in: Nothing. This is my Jewish parents speaking. All they'd say of suffering is, "It always comes back."

Other books tell me one reason why my joints grind and flare: the Thames River vents so much damp into Oxford that even rocks rot. No wonder students look runny and pale, as if sent here expressly to sicken. So in Oxford I can drop any contempt for my clumsy gait. Like the next-door daffodils my depression can all go over to the other side, to plain despair. And what a release it is. For this worsening body of mine at least I'm not to blame.

Now that I've discovered despair, I want to feel its power, which is to say I want to know the worst that's been said of my malady. From an Oxford English Dictionary and a medical glossary I learn the antique terms flinging curses at me: *Arthritis deformans*, the deforming disease, or *Arthritis pauperum*, the aching of the poor. It's hard to imagine what comfort anyone took from the Greek idea of *rheum* (a liquidy swelling), root of *rheumatism*. Looking for more words, I come on Shakespeare's *A Midsummer Night's Dream*: "the moon . . . washes all the air, that rheumatic diseases do abound." And on the frightening phrase "joint-racking Rheums" in Milton's *Paradise Lost*. I find grim eloquence in Thomas Sydenham, a great seventeenth-century physician-writer who favored the notion that rheumatism "takes the joints in turns, and . . . attacks last with redness and swelling." Joints in turns: that's pretty good. I definitely approve of the character in Jane Austen's *Sense and Sensibility* who has a "rheumatic feel in one of his shoulders." And I like the nineteenth-century doctors who put their minds to naming this rheumatic feel. In 1859 Alfred Baring Garrod of London made up "rheumatoid arthritis," a mongrel term—kind of inflammatory, kind of skeletal. Words that disparage my ailment have an oddly elevating effect on me.

If I take a modern definition of rheumatoid arthritis—"a chronic systemic disease, usually polyarticular, marked by inflammatory changes in the synovial membranes, by atrophy, and by rarefaction of the bones"—if I give these words a will of their own, then I hear the flow in *rheumatic*, the ticking of *chronic*, the eloquence of *polyarticular* (any jointed segment), while *atrophy* (the wasting of joints and tendons) means "not to nourish" in Greek, and *rarefaction* (less dense, more fracture prone) sounds like something poet Robert Herrick could have worked with: Then, then, how fragile she has grown / With rarefaction in her bone.

How could I ever have believed this disease had nothing to say for itself? I find even more in the Psalms: "By reason of the voice of my groaning, my bones cleave to my skin." "I am poured out like water, and all my bones are out of joint." In these ancient words my despair sounds recognized.

And later that day this despair even justifies a breathless faith. Our landlord's gardener, all leather patches and good wool, watches me shuffling toward the front gate, head down, spirit down, and announces, "Lovely raspberries you'll have here." Not bloody likely when I'm still in a parka. But July brings a revival that comes and comes again: raspberries, thousands of them, explode off the bushes into our hands.

I'm so unready for this redeeming warmth that I have to buy a cotton dress, sheer and tight. I realize I must be quite thin. And yet my round-cheeked ID photo proves me a pumpkin head. It takes nerve to register the moonface I've been wearing around, from cortisone slipping big deposits of fat into my cheeks. No doubt it's also performing other magic, like ulcerating my stomach and softening my bones. Clearly the disease and its cure are going to get worse, but I didn't make my face lumpy; cortisone did. Clearly it's cockeyed to depend on raspberries for reprieve—but just knowing they always come back, like suffering, frees me up, as a Psalm says, to "taste and see."

A few weeks later, leaving the place where I discovered despair, I take home proof that it pardoned me. My ID photo, looking just plain cheeky in my view, goes on a bedside table, the last soul I see as the light blinks out. Goodnight, Moonface.

Moves, 1994–95

How can a soul rise to the occasion of illness?

I ask the question silently, leaning across a chessboard where Alek's queen is needling my king. Our chess-playing started in England last year, to distract us both.

"Move something," he says, "or you're in check."

I shrug. It's always like this, me playing to stay out of the way.

"Just move."

"What the hell." I try a brazen play, and soon I'm poaching on his pieces.

"Check," says Alek.

My king steps regally to one side.

"Check."

Steps once more.

"You can't go there."

"OK. We're going here."

"And . . . checkmate."

So this is how a person rises to an illness—by stepping away a square at a time, sideswiping as she goes.

"You made some great moves, Ma," Alek says. "See what it feels like to mount an offense? Instead of just reacting to what's going on?"

"Yeah. I do. But I totally lost."

At least now I know what the job is: mount an offense when no match is mine to win. This is going to take some moves.

Move #1. Keeping Track

I've already tried access, steroids, travel. And my joints keep stinging, so what now? It can't hurt to line up a brief log in two columns, to sketch the day's doings, the day's pain, and see if the two sides tie in.

Awful day: Charlotte Salomon	*Pretty pained.*
publicity and midterm exams	
Another awful day: hearing	*Stomach bad too.*
students spew Judeophobia.	

It's no surprise that joint pain goes hand in hand with misery at work. I feel devastated when an artist makes a Malcolm X fresco at San Francisco State's student union, painting Stars of David next to "African blood" and claiming that "Jews owned 75 percent of all slaves." At the same moment, my biography of Charlotte Salomon is being published when I least understand how she survived the lies against Jews. But of course she didn't survive them. For her sake I summon the nerve to speak about the dangers of Judeophobia, but some students only ask, "You believe the Holocaust matters more than other genocides?" as if I'd ever say that. I do say, "The Holocaust *succeeded* beyond any genocide before, killing almost every Jewish gene in Europe, and I've seen this fact denied."

Weeks later I'm slowly crossing my campus when the question comes back to me without Nazis or malice. "You think arthritis matters more than other diseases?" Would I ever say that? It's just that arthritis *succeeds* beyond most ailments, and its monstrousness is disbelieved.

With the fresco fouling my workplace, I move inward to my family. What luck that our daughter Sarah has come back to the Bay Area after college to be a preschool teacher, a profession she took to while working at her brother's daycare. Alek is turning thirteen and teaching clarinet, sometimes to a young Latina, Annette Solo, hoping she takes the name Claire to win fame as Claire Annette Solo. In awe I watch him whipping out a clarinet at his bar mitzvah, blowing a klezmer tune and running the service by himself, just like his sister twelve years before. I hide my campus anxiety so he'll go on thinking it's safe to make a public act of being Jewish.

When the fresco is finally removed, I know its lies have burned me as deeply as joint pain. If the Angel of Anatomy ever offers me a lifetime choice, anti-Semitism or arthritis, I won't turn down my disease.

With this in mind I go back to my two-column experiment, aligning degrees of pain with outside circumstance.

Lovely day: Sarah invites me to lunch.	*Pain.*
Surprise: post-publication reviews of my Charlotte Salmon book.	*Worse.*
Angry and depressed: stupid way to live.	*Worse.*
It's an awful illness, RA.	*Terrible pain.*
Yom Kippur at Stanford with Sarah and John leading songs. Alek throws up from fasting, then reads the Torah before a thousand people.	*Bad aches.*
Wonderful Palo Alto parade with Alek as drum major.	*Joints killing me.*
Great last class, then grading 65 exams. Close to nervous breakdown.	*No words.*
Most relaxed day in months: cooking, buying knee-socks.	*Pain and stumbling.*
First lazy day of 1995. One per annum!	*5 ibuprof. @ a time.*
God. My book won American Historical Association Prize.	*Searing shoulder.*
Weeping about RA. How to live?	*Awful a.m. pain.*
Taking Alek to Honor Band; he nails the solos.	*Ill with pain.*
Must change my life.	——
Very discouraging appointment: M.D. is "shocked."	*16 ibuprofen, no use.*
Alek playing Brahms—how gorgeous.	*14 aspirin: nothing.*
Daylong, nightlong pain.	*Done for.*

As soon as I compare the columns, they prove that awful days ache. But so do handsome days. Apparently my joints don't care what's going on outside. What's more, they give me pain from writing about pain. Stupefied, I shelve my log in favor of finding someone else's.

Move #2. Surveying the Field

There's a book I want to find in the worst way, a book about someone
struck by arthritis and how a life turned out. I try many popular health
books about arthritis but only find doctors speaking to patients, not
the other way around. I scroll through library abstracts, finger-pick
catalogs, looking for a personal account or even a cultural survey of the
disease, and turn up Rosemary Sutcliff's memoir of juvenile arthritis
in England: shut in a ward with one weekly visit, she writes with such
cheer a reader ends up blue. Where are the sufferers who mope and
snort and take it on the chin?

Not in fiction. Maybe social histories? Nothing in the air. I wander
into TB and polio, cancer and AIDS, yellow fever and malaria, plague
and more plague. The voices of suffering make a terrible noise. But
soundlessness is awful too.

Here we have a monstrous malady and no full story from a sufferer
or even *one* account of its long-term impact on human society.

Clearly if lots of writers had given voice to arthritis, I would know
about it, everyone would know about it, arthritis would be acclaimed.
Soundless instead, it's hushing up my own voice too. I decide to collect
fragments in a manila folder, noting whenever the odd writer mentions
my disease—not that they name it. A great poem by Josephine Miles
only calls her RA, suffered since childhood, "a hard life":

> This is a hard life you are living
> While you are young,
> My father said,
> As I scratched my casted knees with a paper knife.
> By laws of compensation
> Your old age should be grand.

By laws of compensation a fine writer shouldn't have arthritis at
all, but here's Thomas Jefferson to John Adams: "Crippled wrists and
fingers make writing slow and laborious." And who else don't we
know about? Grandma Moses painted pictures to relieve her joints.
Raoul Dufy painted them in spite of RA. Sandy Koufax pitched and Joe
Montana quarterbacked in the grip of arthritis.

My slim folder yields a few more piercing poems. There's one by
Jan Glading, actually called "Arthritis," in whose shape I see a spine, in
whose line breaks I hear gasps:

> damn:
> ache
> again
> in
> that
> place
> the
> hands
> can't
> reach
> . . . .
> off-limits
> made
> just
> to keep
> pain in.

The damn ache isn't supposed to be spoken of. From poet Audre
Lorde: "We have been schooled to be secret and stoical about pain
and disease. But that stoicism and silence does not serve us nor our
communities, only the forces of things as they are." Here's Adrienne
Rich, suffering from unnamed rheumatoid arthritis and indicting the
forces of things as they are:

> when the insect of detritus crawls
> from shoulder to elbow to wristbone
> remember: the body's pain and the pain on the streets
> are not the same   but you can learn
> from the edges that blur   O you who love clear edges
> more than anything   watch the edges that blur

These are the deepest words I've ever read on my condition. They
ought to earn any writer a title, like "Articulator of human bones,"
a character in Charles Dickens's *Our Mutual Friend*. What an aim—to

become an Articulator (as in the Latin *articulare*, to make something jointed), connecting and speaking of bones, linking "the body's pain and the pain on the streets."

For me, sadly, every way to articulate bones ruins bones. Just putting trouble into words punishes my arm joints. Should I quit writing? I ought to. Any minute now.

By luck the last sheets in my folder come from two writers facing just this dilemma. So severe was arthritis for Eudora Welty that she had to be carried up stairways. Dropped by accident, she stayed in the hospital a month. Twenty years after she won the Pulitzer Prize, a 1993 interviewer asked whether she was still writing: "No. . . . It is just too physical, writing." Couldn't she tape-record her words? "Now, I can't do that. . . . The page is where I work."

Then the opposite tack comes from Henry Roth's celebrated third-person memoir: "He sat with eyes squeezed shut against the atrocious pain. Every joint in his body, from fingertip to elbow to shoulder," pierced him. How could he bear to write? "Oh, there were tricks in every trade, more than one way to skin a cat, or outwit rheumatoid arthritis." Yes, the craft of writing can "outwit rheumatoid arthritis." And no, "it is just too physical, writing." Like Welty I ought to stop. Like Roth of course I'll keep on.

Move #3. Acting Bold

One day when my arms ache too much to lift a pen, I help my history department interview a high-energy candidate and realize the hidden dilemma inside a hidden handicap—the fear that I'll lose all means to write and they'll wonder why they hired *me*. After the meeting, in the chairperson's office, I come clean: "My joints feel so bad I've got to have an easier schedule . . ."

"That's my job," he says, to my surprise. "Just let me know how to help." Clearly he comes from a kinder planet, but I realize I've never asked my little commonwealth to help me before. What's making me act bolder is watching my colleague Paul Longmore stay up-front about polio in his hands and back. Later, at a campus reception, I grab a seat beside Paul to feed him the best stuff. "A little more pâté?" I ask, my own grip shaky on the cracker. He strengthens *me*. He shows me how people like us could say what disablements we're struggling with.

Confess, and then someone else will, until it's clear we're no cowering minority in the family of humankind.

So let me confess (to myself, for a start): I'm the woman walking to the faculty club with stiff ankles and snapping knees, elbows at right angles, and hands curled up. I'm the woman who can't open the ketchup or the soda bottle or the window blind. I'm the one with the scratchy voice ordering "decaf and large fries," the one with the wispy hair, a side effect of taking methotrexate. It's a strong immune suppressor used against cancer, and did I mention it's scattering strands of hair over the ladies' room sink? That in the mirror I stare at hints of scalp?

In the faculty dining room I scan with envy the tops of female teachers' heads. Their hair seems a primary code they wouldn't feel present without. One has hers dyed and permed, a seeming cover-up of a good hard head. Another wears hers rowed, announcing her descent. Another lets it fly around, resisting what her parents raised. Yet another, hair cut to a brush, looks defiantly at everyone. But start losing this feature females get to fix, and you never want to come out of the ladies' room. You can level with others about anything, but this loss of hair, of woman-power, puts you in disgrace.

I sit down with my fries and recall a friend saying her hardest loss in chemotherapy was just her hair, and now she's rejoicing, smack in the middle of cancer, because the first fuzz has reappeared. Another friend in chemo told me she takes off her scarf at the movies, then walks into the lobby and even into her office just as she is, a grinning woman with ears. Now that's bold. But some of us lose our logo forever, thanks to toxins, menopause, medications, genetics, autoimmunities. Some of us have to choose—but how?—between a need for joints and a need for hair.

My choice comes so abruptly it pushes me up from the table. I decide to stop methotrexate. My doctor wants to keep me on the drug or bump up my cortisone, but I'm dropping them all, disgusted with seeing side effects in the ladies' room mirror.

A month later come the kickbacks, the unleashing of immune cells, as I fall back on antimalarials. The disease steps up, my moonface thins down, and the light-brown marsh grass on my head keeps getting stringier, but not so fast.

Move #4. Setting Defenses

Half a year later it's time to withdraw that move. I do it one day in a group I call Body & Soul (these days my mind's not on my mind). We've joined to sustain a friend whose daughter has died and to talk over tiny troubles of our own. This time I say I've got a problem to solve, and faces brighten: something soluble, imagine that. "Whether to start methotrexate again," I say, "though it can damage the liver. In people like me it strips hair."

"Lots of women in chemo—"

"No. With RA you keep the drug, lose the hair."

These are old friends. They've said I always go the extra mile for them, as much as anyone they know. They used to call me a head-turner when I relied on swinging blond curls and tight poor-boy sweaters, when I mattered because my looks shouted "Hey!" They wished they could trade their own hair for my swishy, not-graying feather-cut. Later they watched me grow unsure of what to count on, humbled by RA. Now I'm choosing to lose the last body part they ever wanted me to swap.

"At some point ahead," I quaver, "would you take me to buy . . . a headscarf?" I can't say *wig*.

"You say when."

"And to lunch?"

"Done."

As soon as kindly women promise *"We'll handle that,"* I realize I won't actually need a headscarf or a wig—and I restart the drug.

But to take these methotrexate pills each week without counting what they take from me, like strands of hair or bits of motherboard, I need to fool my own eyes. Pill dispensers do the trick. They presort a month's medications so I don't spend each breakfast moaning over labels and side effects. The little plastic dispenser pours out a cornucopia of chemicals: yellow methotrexate, lemon folic acid, creamy antimalarials, white ibuprofen, golden vitamin E, chalky calcium from oyster shells. When the morning's dosage spills into my hand, it's like the unlidding of a gem box. At my kitchen table, just for an instant, arthritis colorizes my life.

Move #5. Calculating Costs

In the afternoon I count what that pillbox is worth. Let's see: three methotrexate tablets times four weeks, plus two blood tests, would set me back a hundred bucks, except my insurance takes care of it for five dollars (subtracting hair).

Insurance like mine, says my older brother in New York, doesn't cover jobs like his. He employs himself as a software designer, a world-class chess and bridge master, a wholehearted dad, and a nicotine addict. One night by phone he says he's in the hospital for urgent surgery. I'm not asked to help, but all the same I'm terrified my non-insured brother will need my savings—college for Alek, support for Sarah, work leaves for my joints—or else he'll die. But what actually happens suits his style (play the cards) better than mine (do this? do that?). Apparently hospital orderlies lift him onto a burning-hot sterilized gurney, and he announces he'll sue like Satan. I imagine some mainframe voids his bills before they're even sent out.

My brother recovers, but I'm still stuck in doctors' waiting rooms, logging instructional hours. One day I daydream a new facility, a health college for both the chronics and the acutes (my brother's team). The receptionist over there would register us for physical therapy, pain management, addiction control, and more. Tuition would come from taxpayers who know if we molder at home now, we'll need big-ticket care later. A reference shelf would tell of countries where taxation spreads health costs throughout the public, unlike this country, where private insurance hands off the bill to employers, employees, spouses, sisters. If taxpayers complained ("We're already paying for Medicare and Medicaid. Now health college too?"), the patients who calculate costs would reply, "It's a steal."

Move #6. Anticipating Losses

"However do you manage?" a graduate student asks me across my office desk.

I feel a squall of fury that I manage by paying in cash and time—if not for healthcare, then for every task. "My last memo to you ('Reminder of our meeting Tuesday') required a mike, a typist, a payment, a week's wait, a revision . . ."

98

GETTING BACK

"Tedious," agrees the student softly.

"It's like writing by intravenous drip. You know, I used to live for fingertip communication. Now I live as if it's not invented yet."

"I don't see how you stand it."

"Well . . ." I scratch for some compensation. "Now that I can't dash off my own letters to friends, I get on the phone. Now that I don't pencil students' papers, I make the comments face to face. And I like it. I like talking." I'm warming to this. "To everyone who relies on writing I'd say, Oral culture has its uses. It's good to hear your voice again."

Convincing as this sounds, I sneak back to the written word by way of DragonDictate, a 1995 computer program paid for by state disability so I can do my job at half the cost of paying scribes. Speech recognition, I'm forewarned, is a whole new ball and chain. My colleague Paul prefers writing on his stomach with a mouth pen and ventilator to using that software. But I mince ahead and abruptly flunk to remedial. My every phrase turns mushy in the circuitry. And a worse trap waits ahead.

Just when I shift to software, this voice-intensive program takes away my voice. It isn't laryngitis. It's my vocal cords straining too much for arthritis. As far as I know, I've blown the essential moving part, with no more hope for its return than for agile hands.

I become a proverbial silent woman, moving my mouth in pantomime. No way will I talk via notes, because my hands can't write them, and for the same reason I'll never learn signing. So nothing greets my son Alek except "Have a great day," mouthed in the morning, and "How was your day?" when he's home from high school. The hardest moment comes one night at the kitchen table when Alek starts on free speech—the harm of hate words versus the insult of censorship—a subject so close to my cortex I can feel it bulging behind my eyes. I say nothing, of course, but for me the end of free speaking is the end of being. And I can't pass a word of this to anyone. Silently I retrace this year's tactics against RA: keep track, survey the field, act bold, set defenses, calculate costs, anticipate losses. This loss I didn't anticipate.

But if there's one thing I've learned with RA, it's to feel completely done for and then give it another month. In that month my problem reaches friends, and consolations arrive I never guessed at. One-way phone calls and notes I can't answer pour in. Drowsy bedtime talks with John, a habit of thirty years, go by the board, but I find him staying awake to look my way. He takes a long moment to kiss me, inhaling my whole day's unsaid words, along with a little bit of my tongue, while a night owl hoots a steady pulse, a sound I intend to make soon. The next morning squirrels chitter, and more gifts arrive. From my friend Ruth comes a flashcard ("Please Understand. I Can't Talk Now"), and from my friend Mary a textile I deck the computer with, delighted to demote my machinery to drapery. Then my doctor starts a drop-dead course of cortisone that finally locates my vocal cords, while a speech pathologist trains them to make soft sounds ("Shape words with lips, send air through lungs"). I try this on John's mouth until we're sputtering.

All my words have moved from manual to vocal to facial and now settle where I have to quit saying them whenever a radio's on or a dish-washer's running or a van's going by, where I wait for a noiseless house before I dial my daughter, where a hissing faucet stops me midphrase and I mike conversations that aren't one-on-one. Inside this subdued place, just short of speechlessness, I live in permanent check—and plot how to put off the endgame.

Truths, 1996

Move by move I play against this condition of mine, never winning, but mounting an offense—my son's advice over a chessboard—instead of letting things happen. Then in the midst of my moves I come upon a confounding truth.

Browsing a local health newsletter for some swimming-pool hours, I spot a column calling arthritis "an unrecognized major women's health problem," affecting twenty-three million American women. I scribble: "Swim Friday noon. Twenty-three million?" The newsletter, quoting the Centers for Disease Control and Prevention, the federal CDC, probably hiked the number. I better track it down.

The next morning, from the depths of Stanford Medical Library, I bring out the CDC's *Morbidity and Mortality Weekly Report*, surveying sickness unto death every seven days. Recent 1995 issues disclose something I don't think many people know. Arthritis is "the leading cause of disability" in the U.S. population over age sixty-five, attacking every second senior citizen—but not just seniors. Well before the age of fifty half the population shows signs of arthritis. Across all ages the full disease goes after 15 percent of the populace. It forms "a leading cause of work-related disability in the United States." Work-related. People in their prime.

It's also the "leading cause of activity limitation" stinting the lives of women, the ailment women themselves blame before anything, even before cancer or heart disease.

As medical statistics go, these numbers are stunning. The disease is a national curse. Yet it's lived inside my joints for a quarter-century without my measuring the breadth of it.

Picking a few articles, I set out for our place in the Santa Cruz Mountains, ready to size up some truths. Once there, though, I have to deal with drought. Knobcone pines and Douglas fir are losing needles, and the begonias I planted in memory of my dad's terrace look crisped. I drag a hose to a knobcone, then slip back to the sofa where my articles are spread. After an hour I'm sure of one thing.

The diseases called arthritis batten on my sex.

Of course I've always noticed that my doctor's waiting area resembles a ladies' locker room. But now I'm finding evidence from the Arthritis Foundation that arthritis strikes women over men two to one. One-third of women between the ages of forty-five and sixty-four have some kind of arthritis, as do more than half of women over sixty-five. Nodules from arthritis, sometimes quite painful, appear only in women. And arthritis limits women's activities twice as severely as men's (even adjusting for female longevity). Also, three-quarters of those with autoimmune diseases (RA among them) are women. Some scientists say autoimmune diseases could be "teleologically related to the female's reproductive function" since "no biological system is developmentally more important to the female than the capability to reproduce."

Well, bite that story. Developmentally, reproduction isn't "more important to the female." It is important to the species. Autoimmune diseases land harder on women because humanity wants to survive and watches half of itself pay.

I change the hose over to an oak tree, then go back to the sofa. Take Americans with osteoarthritis, the most common kind. Osteoarthritis falls everywhere, on both women and men, but sixteen of twenty-one million serious sufferers are female, and over age forty-five women get it worse and live with it longer. In any of its forms arthritis creates the leading chronic problem for women in mid- and later life, and it's women who have "notably higher rates of difficulty" with movement, strength, endurance.

Then there's the worst kind, rheumatoid. A solid two-thirds to three-quarters of RA patients are women. And women suffer the severest cases. As for age, RA clusters in females age thirty-five to fifty-five but often begins around twenty-five and even attacks thousands of youngsters.

A pause to pull the hose slowly to the begonias, which are falling apart, bud from stem. No way, I whisper, will you crumble on my watch. I turn up the flow, the way my dad watered.

Here's the clincher for a feminist: the CDC confesses, "The public-health importance of arthritis among women has not been emphasized." Start with the fact that "female excess in incidence has been apparent for many years," at all ages, yet only a few studies "even verify the age and gender findings." I can guess why researchers don't often bother. One thing we rely on is a busy woman never getting crippled up. Who would fill in for her, lifting babies, mashing potatoes, cleaning cafeterias, grading papers, doing all the jobs nobody picks up after? It's easier to ignore arthritis than to face the fact that it preys on women in their prime.

This avoidance has hushed me up for years. This notion that women's tasks are indispensable and women's pains bearable has swaddled me and fleeced me.

Am I wrong about the muting of women's complaints? Looking again at rheumatic and autoimmune ailments, I see cultural interest excited by gout (one of the more treatable forms), once linked to masculine excess, tapping men over women seven to one. Meanwhile rheumatic diseases with low profiles follow the secondary status of their mostly female sufferers. RA hits four females for every male, while lupus goes after five women (some researchers say fifteen) for every man, among them a writer I love, Flannery O'Connor. To the begonias again. She was killed by it. Sofa again. Sleep.

In the dry afternoon I wake to pop open pill bottles, a pricier sound than women's old-time pain relief, their dripping poultices and patting of pillows. For tablets to whisk away suffering, Americans in the 1990s spent three billion dollars a year. By myself I account for $2000 in medicine and another $2000 to see the doctor (both covered by good insurance), then add the huge cost of not working full-time, of having to hire household help, of paying a typist $100 for each job, and I'm up to $12,000 a year. Women—and it's mostly women—who fall below the poverty line can't afford my way of having arthritis. They endure it below the line for treating pain.

It's unthinkable how many of them have my elbows minus my income, how many worsen with "low income and lack of personal freedom" (read: female lives). It's easier for a society to blink when only a quarter of disabled women find work, only half of disabled men, easier to overlook the elbow-grease jobs hurting female joints or to skip the fact that arthritis grows two times worse for African Americans and three times more frequent for people earning less than $10,000 a year.

I check my notes one last time to get this straight: how does the CDC explain these dreadful differences? "The reasons for higher rates of arthritis among women and higher rates of activity limitation among women and persons with low education and low income are . . ."— holding my breath—"not clear."

Knowing *who* is struck, but not why, comes as a shock that calls for true-life stories—maybe even mine. I head outside and shut off the tap, too shaken to stay longer and soak more plants. The drought gets to win after all.

At home, in our backyard, I tell John the disheartening truth that connective-tissue diseases like RA and osteoarthritis, lupus and multiple sclerosis, all stick it harder to women.

"Does it help much to know this?"

"It helps so much I have to think why." It takes me a moment to turn his question over. I've seen arthritis as a curse, I realize, one reserved for me by the Angel of Anatomy in exchange for others: so Alek and Sarah wouldn't fall ill and lose their knack for rocketing down swimming lanes, so John wouldn't have his dad's heart attacks, so my own dad wouldn't pass through pain, so Ruth wouldn't perish from breast cancer, so I wouldn't get cancer too. Now I know the Angel swoops over my whole half of the human race. Grasping this does make all the difference: arthritis isn't just a hardship now, it's an issue. I turn to John. "Breast cancer became an issue when activists made a national fuss, and officials started paying attention to the female vote."

"They *know* breast cancer goes with being female."

"Right. And arthritis does too—a fact that isn't so known." It's like other problems—poverty, illiteracy, starvation—that decimate women before anyone else. Because improving the welfare of women is a swift way to reduce human suffering, it's clear why arthritis ought to be a humanist and feminist cause. But is it?

I try my luck in the field of women's health, where fresh 1990s titles range from sexuality to cancer to bias against body parts, but not a peep about the disease that hurts so many females. It seems feminism leaves an attention deficit as deep as the public one. McGraw-Hill's fifty-nine reprints on female health manage one *page* about arthritis, from a household magazine. I'm impressed to see breast cancer made public, but where's my cohort on joints? Of course arthritis doesn't take life, but it does radiate enough heat to confuse a thermostat and merit a story or two. Maybe we're so busy denying women are the weaker sex we don't admit women are the sicker sex—not sick with arthritis anyway.

Personally my hands are full already, pressing women's studies on my university, moving gender into a view of genocide, teaching history that places each body inside bonds of gender and ethnicity, of income and sexuality. I'm not ready for broadcasting arthritis as a female ailment, and here's another reason why. "Right now rheumatoid arthritis attacks two and a half million Americans," I tell my friend Ruth, "and since they're mostly women, I'm *scared*."

I'm scared of any malady that discriminates by sex: ovarian cancer, cervical cancer, breast cancer (which Ruth knows as well as her face), autoimmune ailments, and arthritis, which mostly strikes our gender without anyone knowing exactly why.

All this scares Ruth too, but not much else does. Seven years past cancer and doing fine, she often says, like Audre Lorde, "After cancer, what's there to be afraid of?" (Except cancer again.)

A few months later, in the grip of a flareup, I confide to Ruth's answering machine, "My doctor says he's shocked again. Phone when you can."

Later that night she calls: "I saw my doctor too." Then a long silence. "It's primary breast cancer again."

On two ends of the phone line she cries and I cry and she cries. What is *happening*? Why would the Angel of Anatomy send cancer again and ratchet up RA?

Early the next morning John and I rush to Berkeley to talk with Ruth, who already has a strategy: surgery, right away. Afterward she awakens in hospital and is told, Go home now, you're only covered for one day. What exactly should she do that night at home—throw a bash? All she

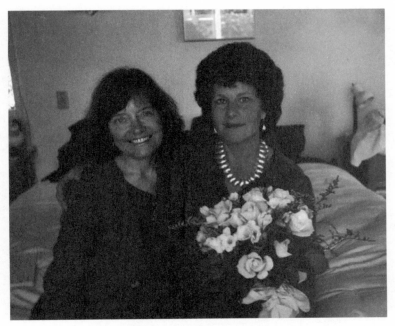

Mary and Ruth, 1996. Photo courtesy of the author.

can do is repeat her own advice, which her quick heart passes on to me: "A disease looks bad. Still, you don't know for sure. Be an agnostic."

Be an agnostic about your own case, but take for certain one prime truth. Getting Ruth's disease or mine is not—as I wanted it to be, wishing the Angel of Anatomy flew blind—simply not, for our gender, hit-or-miss.

Pieces, 1996–97

If I ask women, Does my day remind you of yours? more hands might go up than I ever imagined. My day starts with cursing the icebox for making me hoist my arms. It continues at the office with unbending my joints on my mother's old yoga pad, then rocking like a turtle, trying to rise. Driving home after classes gives me creaks in the neck, then John's welcoming hug hurts my shoulders. And that's a good day.

"Every joint's a royal pain," is all I can say—a pain in the neck, the wrists, the knees, feet, ankles, elbows, shoulders, hips, and this is just a gross list. If John ever pulls a tendon or strains his back, I feel pity but pass up the chance to identify. I've had days when I can't count the joints that hurt, when it's easier to number the joints that don't.

For anyone in this predicament a time arrives when the most prized activities collapse in the middle. One day, doing a slide show on Charlotte Salomon in a Harvard lecture hall where I took notes thirty-five years before, I'm expressing an excited desire to write another biography. Then that desire goes rip. I can hardly make it off the podium. My joints are signaling: No traveling around anymore, scurrying to archives, roving for interviews, lifting document boxes. After the talk I tell myself, It's *over*. Biographer, historian, can-do researcher—that whole former life is cutting me loose. Over the next days uncertainty makes me take a step for the first time. I put my body's trouble on tape:

> All morning I'm dropping with fatigue. What if I worked
> an assembly line where falling asleep I'd get maimed?
> (Pause tape.)
> Now it's noon and the joints reach high influenza, like
> those weather inversions driving heat closer, unable to
> rise. Anywhere I sit stays hot after I get up. I open a

magazine and words simmer away, then it slips off my
thumbs. (Pause tape.)
Late afternoon, my heat inversion lifts. I see friends. They
say I look good. Just before sleep, I wave away what
will come a few hours later. This disease gives wicked
meaning to the words *double life*. (Off.)

A week later I tell my friend Adele, who has flown from Chicago to
see me, "I'm too ashamed to hand this tape to a typist I hardly know—"
"But I want to *read* it," Adele interrupts.
Whatever for? I check with my friend Joan in New Jersey. "Are daily
pains worth reading about?"
She laughs. "Try Nancy Mairs on multiple sclerosis." That afternoon
I have every book by Mairs on the library table in front of me. With grace
she writes of limbs that never look or work the way they're supposed
to. She copes with MS "by speaking about it, and about the whole
experience of being a body, specifically a female body, out loud."
Invited just then to join a San Francisco writing group, my first time
among writers of great experience, I'm moved to pump up a project or
two—not a big biography again, I'm sad to say, but maybe a little piece
about the "experience of being a body" with my ailment, you know, uh,
arthritis. I start to mention its lack of status in medicine and culture,
when phhtt! the idea deflates: too hard on my arms. "I shouldn't join
your group. I'm not so much a writer anymore."
Silence. Then they all jump in, surprised their craft is so tough on
joints, curious why I call arthritis a "medical mystery" or "cultural
blank," amazed I can fancy tiptoeing around it. They think I'll have
to push straight through. Could I start with a little explanatory tape
recording for my teenage son? And not, they stress, get hung up on
writing?
On their thermals alone I swoop down the freeway from San Francisco. Right here I have something to put on tape: a day in the life of
my joints. As an open letter to my son then? No, an unopened one. At
night I talk into my tape recorder for five embarrassed minutes about
my body. A few days later ten minutes. The cassette winds forward in
little speech-bursts, starting with, "Alek, you always hear clumps (my
right foot down a stair) and pauses (left one catching up). You always

hear, Hey, could you take this box upstairs for me? And do me a favor,
bring my backpack down?" and ending with, "I mean it, I was sturdy till
this disease came to me, about twelve years before *you* did. But that's a
story for some other day . . ."

Weeks later I take my unopened letter to the writers' group, which
listens and makes a collective comment: "Sure, your body's in pieces,
but your mind is gluing it together."

When John asks later, "What are you taping there?" I say, "Little
mismatched pieces, like legs and arms glued onto Mr. Potato Head."

I keep tape-recording till we take off for a month-long residency at
the Rockefeller Center on Lake Como, where John's translating German and Spanish poetry. Among its artists and scholars I read some
pieces aloud, abashed that no one stands to learn from aching joints.
But over the next days, to my surprise, listeners nudge me into corners
to tell me about their own beleaguered bodies. My God, people carry
secret suffering around.

What makes anyone ever bring it out? For an answer I'm reading Ken-
neth Fries's *Body, Remember*: "As our bodies begin to fail, . . . emotions
long stored beneath the skin, within our bones, are released." But
released how?

I hear my officemate's keyboard go click-click, and a tingling startles my fingertips, estranged from any keyboard for years. Suddenly
they manage to recall a Smith Corona, "Syncopated Clock," a Bach
harpsichord suite. "But my mind doesn't remember any of that," I say.

After a moment Toni asks, "How did Holocaust survivors you inter-
viewed retrieve their memories?"

"Well, it's odd. They used disclaimers like 'I can't remember' or 'I'm
not sure anymore,' which I skipped over, to highlight facts. One day I
reversed the highlighting, just looked at the disclaimers, and noticed
these captured a deeper pain, that they couldn't get their hands on
truth."

"Try that," she says.

"Try reverse-highlighting? Make use of what my conscious effort
won't remember?" Instantly I think of my mother, mobile as long as
her legs told her how to walk instead of her mind.

That's when I get the idea to reverse-highlight the "whole experience of being a body" (in Nancy Mairs's words), to remember from the body to the mind. Actually it's the body pushing me to try this. One evening after a long workday my right ankle turns so falling-down painful that it quits bearing weight. John saves me by digging out my father's walking stick, and I make it around the house feeling like Old Lady with Cane, a dreaded icon of my disease.

On the other hand, what timing. The next day I'm scheduled to go where a cane's an entrance badge, a disability conference featuring Nancy Mairs, who says an autoimmune disease "weights your whole body with a weariness no amount of rest can relieve. An alien invader must be at work. But of course it's not. It's your own body. That is, it's you." At the conference I wanted to air the "you" I've kept bunched behind my ordered self like a raggedy towel.

But I never get to show I belong there, because the next day I can't walk on either ankle. Too disabled for the disability conference. Not disabled enough to prepare for this standstill.

All afternoon I fret about bad ankles #1 and #2. What will I get around on? Crutches? Out of the question: they require weight-bearing wrists. Cane? My fingers can't grip hard enough to hold me up.

What is it with these joints? Is the person they belong to—me? These two-bit questions, to my surprise, fetch up returns. I used to say of the past, "I'm not sure anymore." But when I reverse-highlight, illuminating not the action but the ankles that carried the action, suddenly its essence bursts open. At age eight those ankles were dancing "Sorcerer's Apprentice" with abandon, in brown felt rhythm slippers, and at age seventeen they were prancing in high heels around a laboratory. Yes, that's who I was—I'd forgotten. If I just let a body part cue my mind, it lifts to light the person no longer visible, the one before the one who now takes pains to place her feet.

With ankles wrapped in hot-pads, I have nowhere to go but history. From an afternoon with a cane comes my best scheme yet for gluing mind and motion together. *Think back through the joints.*

Wonder, 1941–49

As my ankles grow a bit stronger, I think back to an earlier life that shaped my handling of illness, to earlier skills and warnings I never brought into alignment before. Medical treatments never reached this one thing I can do for myself. They scan present symptoms and then leave off before tapping the renewable energy of memory. Joint memory brings out events and currents my body has responded to, ideas of health and illness that ran through me since childhood, lessons in living, especially living female, picked up from those years.

Remembering the early years would be easier if someone had bothered to write "Arthritis before You Got It: 1940s to 1960s," but no such luck. I'll have to go after the vital questions on my own.

Who was I before I ran into the disease?

What was the disease before it ran into me?

For material I ask John to take down from the attic some boxes I found in Pittsburgh after my parents died. Going through them, postcard by photo, diary by notebook, I discover the ruling myths I've held about my pre-arthritis years. Always I've felt certain my parents worked hard to improve my mind, while I worked on my body. But evidence from the 1940s shows it was the other way around. In my memory of the fifties I never had goals beyond boyfriends, but the boxes prove I had brainy ambitions all along, trusting mental effort to shape my body and life. By another ruling myth I had no concern for pain till the morning I woke with burning wrists. I bet this won't turn out to be the case either.

As I spend my evenings looking through the boxes, and my days reading medical history, something curious comes about. Any painful limb I focus on seems stuffed with messages from the time before RA. With this new finding-device I go about cracking a life history joint by joint. The outlines of an earlier self emerge, one headed for nothing like sickness yet used to the idea, believing health was bound to give out. And this suspended sentence owed to growing up exactly when and where I did.

One thing born in 1941, aside from me, was Wonder Woman, the cartoon, and my coming to life that year probably brought the same comic relief. Back then my father had a nightly habit of reading my mother the Pittsburgh papers with their worsening news. Around the night my older brother was born in November 1938, called Kristallnacht in Germany, my parents read of Nazis smashing Jewish property and dragging thirty thousand Jews to torture camps. So the wonder of my birth is that after two more years of news like that they went ahead and had another Jewish child.

Looking back on that time, I realize the early baby boom of my birth took place during the war, not after it, in a moment of defeat, not victory. Jews were being called crooked to the bone, a threat to the "body of European nations," in need of "special treatment," and these charges of "disease" brought sentences of death. Even in America my parents felt they had to raise a healthy child.

So my first memory is of being sent at age three to a day camp where all activities had one theme: eat. Even camp songs pushed the idea of staying safe from danger:

> I don't want to march in the infantry (feet mark time)
> Ride in the cavalry (knees post)
> Shoot with the artillery (hands trigger) . . .

Singing this, I worked up a certain fear that feet, knees, hands could end in harm. Even "Dem Bones, Dem Bones" signaled the trickiness of being jointed: "Hip bone's connected to the thighbone, thighbone's connected to the knee bone, knee bone's connected to the foot bone," only by the word of the Lord.

How did my parents make sure those bones stayed intact? They told me swimming was required, like brushing my teeth or taking baths. By age seven I whip-kicked long laps each afternoon at the Y—the Young Men's Hebrew Association—and afterward leapfrogged the trough of disinfectant and skipped through the shower room, until my swiftness caught me four blocks from home. I hadn't stopped to pee, and now it was running into my stockings. At dusk I arrived soaked and icy, but my parents never fussed because the main thing was to swim.

Swimming seemed its own reward, if you counted the Clark Bar afterward. But for my parents swimming meant crossing from foreign to homegrown, adopting water as a cure-all. Immigrant raised, they'd moved from Yiddish to English, replaced cholent with hot dogs and prayer with reading, but neither of them had built up muscle mass. Even my dad, who "did crew" at college, was the weightless guy calling stroke counts. It was up to his children to break into society through sport. I went to the Y most afternoons because my parents were trying to titrate exactly the mix of muscle and mind that makes a good American. Years later, to preserve that mix, I concealed RA however I could.

At seven, in '49, I asked my mother, "Are they doggy-paddling?" as I flipped through one of her art books. She put on glasses for Lucas Cranach: "They're swimming in the Fountain of Youth." But I saw more than swimming going on. I saw the crippled and sick falling into water and springing out for private snacks and—naps? One lesson wasn't lost on me in my tadpole years: the sick are grotesque, but water puts them right.

Now as I backstroke across the sunny pool at Stanford, I recall the forties' sanctions on swimming, as if it could pollute as well as cure. No swimming outdoors "because of polio." No swimming in Highland Park because it refused Blacks, and none at the nearby Pittsburgh Athletic Association "because our kind," my parents said, "aren't allowed." At that early age I realized a body in water becomes a reflection of faith, of race, of health. As I frog-kicked the widths of the Y, I found out who I was not going to be: Christian or colored or crippled. All those distinctions flowed from postwar Pittsburgh without any effort on my part.

My effort went into make-believe, telling dreamy stories in my room, cribbing phrases from the radio, like "pop foul" and "polio summer" and "sex hormones." This last phrase I didn't quite get, but by third grade I did find boys too chummy, and begged the teacher to push them back.

"They like you, Mary."

"I don't care. Get them away."

At recess they galloped over the playground, while our space was the jungle gym—a few square yards and some altitude. Our trick was to hook ankles under the top rung, then turn upside down till our underpants caught the sun. Trusting my knee bone to stay connected to my thighbone, I thought every joint of my body made me a girl. It was a notion I retained somehow, with the long result that losing the use of my joints felt like falling from femaleness.

Boys, my older brother proved, were a handful and might become wayward youths at Pittsburgh's Child Guidance Center, where my mother served on the board. Naturally I made sure to be the good child she returned to after meetings. Our local pediatrician Dr. Benjamin Spock assured her that a good child, left free to follow a good doctor's advice, would grow healthy and fearless.

But fear got hold of me from the day when third-graders sat cross-legged in the school auditorium to watch a film about the war. As Allied soldiers cleared a concentration camp, a teacher explained briskly that the stick figures shoveled over each other "had been Jews." All at once my knees locked in isosceles, because it seemed those sunken bodies would drown my buoyant one. Escaping from school, I told my mother I'd seen a horror film, and she shot back, "You're safe, you *are*," which set off doubts.

This memory, fixed deep inside my joints, tells me how early I stiffened with fear and how keenly I disbelieved being safe. All the threats to well-being learned in my youngest years (when I was warned to eat, sent into segregated water, shown the war and the bones of Jews) added up to something like knowing—knowing the job in life is to keep the body guarded, for it can meet with harm.

Decades later, memories of myself in the forties come back literally by accident. One day in the Stanford hills my right ankle buckles over a stone, collapsing me near an ancient tree I call Endurance. While my friend Margo stands shocked, I'm stunned by instant recall, as if twisting my ankle opens a turnstile to the past. An image from the third grade comes to me: I'm wearing my favorite ankle socks to match my sweater (a touch of class), while older girls have gone on to bobby socks, then knee-socks, then nylons leading up to garter belts, a sign of readiness. If my ankles stay strong, they'll take me all that way.

Now that they're cueing memory, I recall how else I knew these body parts mattered. On a third-grade field trip to Pittsburgh's Carnegie Museum we visited an archaeologist sorting dinosaur skeletons. When he fitted together two Jurassic digits, my hair stood on end as I imagined them grasping prey. In just that moment I'd grasped joints. This memory comes back so strongly that I look up dinosaurs and discover "the oldest and most widespread pathological lesion reported in paleopathology": arthritis. It's not my singular self getting stiffed. It's a dinosaur disease in my bones. With my fingers stretched toward a window, I see ancient talons, and my little yelp of pain echoes the bellow of triceratops.

This long view of joints brings me to historian Joan Brumberg's "deceptively simple question: What can we learn from the historical study of a particular disease?" What I want to learn is whether RA, a centuries-old form of ancient arthritis, causes as much suffering now as it used to. And why arthritis, and in particular rheumatoid arthritis, has left so little imprint on historical memory. This means finding personal accounts, rare as they are. "Rheumatoid arthritis," wrote suffragist Lydia Becker in 1890, "cripples my limbs and undermines my strength. My physician says he can get me no hope of effective cure." (Her best drug would have been willow bark, eventually pressed into aspirin.) "My elbows and shoulders were . . . suddenly welded into one painful mass by some diabolical trickster," wrote Mary Dietel, years before I knew of RA. "In great pain, I wanted to shout, 'Cut it out, I want peace!' But . . . there is no peace," wrote Pearson Corbett of "the enemy arthritis." Faith Perkins felt "drafted" by RA into a "scattered, battered army . . . that doesn't sleep at night, longing for the day, that gets through the day wishing for the night," a grim life sentence. RA is still dreadful, but at least I've made it past that past. And these sources provide clues: a disease so incurable couldn't fit into popular recovery narratives. It bore cultural fears of being irredeemable.

The "deceptively simple question" of a disease's history keeps me looking further. Was there a decisive shift in irredeemable RA, a moment when modern medicine first took a specific shot at it? What I discover: one signal moment not only changed my disease but altered human health.

When I was young, arthritis in all forms still dissolved in everyday life, as "present" as I was in third-grade homeroom. I remember a bent-up neighbor who hardly knew what to complain of, calling arthritis "the aches." Like black lung (an unspecified condition my parents described before officials admitted its existence) arthritis stayed vague because no one was committed to removing it from workaday life. Government surveys at the time showed it caused more disability, put more people on the dole, than any other condition, so it was not in any sense an obscure disease—just familiar and obscured. No charity collected for it, no federal grant funded it, no new drug worked on it. Almost no doctors specialized in it, no medical training took it up. Even Dr. Harry Margolis, a family friend who pioneered an arthritis clinic in Pittsburgh, never mentioned it in our dining room.

Decades later this early rheumatologist writes to my later one, discussing treatments for me. I remind Dr. B. that Dr. Margolis trained at the only rheumatology program before my time, the Mayo Clinic, under Philip Hench. I ask him, "Do you know much of Dr. Hench?" He laughs and recalls an early film where a patient winces visibly as the great 1940s clinician moves her limbs. "Med students nicknamed him Hench the Wrench."

I walk out of the clinic holding an invisible thread from Dr. B. back to Dr. Margolis to Dr. Hench to Ralph Pemberton, the founding American rheumatologist, who learned the subject in the nation's largest medical laboratory—World War I. Pemberton's early report on 450 soldiers listed their real names and races (always white), plus one thing he couldn't explain: their joints worsened so much they couldn't fight. His verdict: "Chronic arthritis constitutes one of the outstanding medical conditions affecting the soldiering service." It's true: 92,633 American soldiers suffered from this disease in 1917–18, some catching rheumatic fever (from streptococcus, triggering joint and heart disease) and a third picking up osteo or rheumatoid. Apparently their joints couldn't "march in the infantry, ride in the cavalry," as my old camp song said, and stay in working order.

Surrounded by early sources, I give the disease more than my usual grudging attention. In the twenties it became part of an immense cause—namely, to find a cure for arthritis in pursuing an end to war. A farsighted Netherlands physician, Jan van Breemen, tried to bring rival nations into a League against Rheumatism, but after 1918 Americans weren't joining anything called a league, and by 1940 the league's records had vanished, as Germany crushed van Breemen's country in a new world war. By then rheumatic fever was killing more American children each year than polio did in a decade. New sulfa drugs rose to the rescue, inspiring the Navy to dose six hundred thousand sailors in 1943 and touch off a vicious cycle: sulfa-resistant bacteria slipped into undosed bases and ran wild.

Servicemen on crutches because of *arthritis*? Because they had "one of the most disabling" diseases the War Department ever named? Even its cost was staggering: thirty-five thousand disability checks went to arthritic World War I veterans in the midst of World War II; five thousand severe cases entered the Army and Navy Rheumatism Center in '44–45, one-third with RA. The center's director discharged this third from service, then rooted out "psychogenic rheumatism" imitating RA, ordered patients to shun "crutch-psychology," and sent "slightly rheumatic joints" back to the front. This director was Hench the Wrench.

Philip Hench had a sharp eye for RA, observing "within every rheumatoid patient" what he called "corrective forces." These emerged during pregnancy or jaundice and consisted of some "anti-rheumatic substance" flowing from the adrenal glands. In 1941 word spread of adrenals extracted from Argentine cattle to help German pilots fly higher, and then our side supported hormone extraction too. That rumor (false) jump-started arthritis research in this country, along with a brilliant clinician, a crippled fighting force, and a brace of world wars.

Once the Axis fell, Dr. Hench sized up his other foe, then headed to Minnesota's Mayo Clinic. There he trained the Pittsburgh rheumatologist I later consulted (as if consulting Hench), and there he tried an adrenal fix on a woman bedridden with RA. A miracle took place, the signal moment itself: the patient flexed her joints and went "downtown for three hours." Before the fix his other RA patients stumbled through set-up obstacles; after it they jumped over. In 1949 Dr. Hench pronounced rheumatoid arthritis "reversible" and unveiled a wonder drug to the world. He gave it the crisp name of *cortisone*.

I'm spellbound to read a 1949 *Harper's Magazine* claiming that cortisone could handle not only RA but anything from itching to schizophrenia. In the same year, a classic medical text included word of *auto*immune reactions (the kind that treated "self" as "nonself"), for now bodies with autoimmune RA had a mighty steroid defense.

But "our first patient," Dr. Hench's bedridden woman who skipped downtown, needed higher doses all the time. She gained a pound a day, lost it just as fast, showed a "rounding of facial contour," stopped having periods. The doctors also noted fats glomming onto the torso, skin thinning down, bones losing minerals, minds growing manic. I'm reminded of myself before quitting steroids a few years ago, pacing the house with razor-sharp senses, sniffing apples John left out, counting faces on Alek's walls (sixteen of Beatles, one of Brahms), waking in midnight panics. Now I search for reports from cortisone patients in the early days and find them deeply skeptical. Pearson Corbett of Utah, fighting RA with molar extractions, kerosene, and bee stings, finally tried two weeks of cortisone and felt restored to life; then the serum from hog glands ran out, and he suffered *more* than before. The same serum made Flannery O'Connor of Georgia write, "If pigs wore garments I wouldn't be worthy to kiss the hems of them," but it wasn't enough to keep her alive. Mrs. Dick McCoy of Maine said her doctor "weren't doing me no good, giving me that cortisone . . . and I ain't been back to him since for arthritis." Mary Dietel of Tennessee tried potato peelings and bee venom against RA, then bought a little cortisone ("I was eating gold"), which caused ulcers, blurred vision, itching sores. At last she asked doctors if getting off cortisone was "as bad as quitting dope." They said, "Much worse."

These stories bring back what I knew firsthand in the early cortisone days, when I was told that my uncle Abe suffered from a rare disorder and "owed his life" to that steroid. Every weekend I used to visit him and his dogs ("Mopper" and "Mopper's Seeing-Eye"), who summered, my uncle told me deadpan, at Camp Bow-Wow. To me this story seemed as plausible as owing your life to a wonder drug. Soon both dogs were guiding their master around, for my funniest relative lost his sight and puffed up and turned magenta from cortisone. It saved his life. It ruined his health.

Back then Uncle Abe used to say, "Hats off to the companies," though this remark failed to floor me, since I didn't know Syntex and Upjohn were converting Mexican yams into cortisone, making the synthesized drug affordable to him. He rooted for private firms because state-run health, he claimed, along with the whole American Medical Association, would make doctors "slaves of socialism." As our country waged the Cold War on the terrain of health, the steroid miracle, propelled by RA, won a victory for our body politic. Capitalism the theory, medicine the practice, cortisone the proof.

Putting this postwar story together, I realize our cortisone moment came out of a larger trend, forgotten now, when "the aches" of arthritis rose to a modern disease. In one decade of the forties an American researcher isolated "rheumatoid factor," an International Congress on Rheumatic Diseases met for the first time in New York, the Arthritis and Rheumatism Foundation took form under Floyd Odlum (an entrepreneur with RA), a National Arthritis and Rheumatism Act pledged the "rehabilitation of those who have been victims of these diseases," a National Institute of Arthritis and Metabolic Diseases sprouted within the National Institutes of Health, a wonder drug came into being, and a Nobel Prize arrived for Dr. Hench. Transforming an aches-and-pains ailment looked like midcentury man's great game.

My notes pile into this conclusion, but I don't buy it. Arthritis was brought up-to-date by women too. From a forgotten researcher, Eleanor Venning, came proof that adrenal hormones soar during pregnancy. From this proof, and from pregnant patients, emerged the clues to RA remission, clues that led Dr. Hench to cortisone. From Mary Lasker and a pressure group ("Mary and her little lambs") grew the federal Arthritis and Rheumatism Act and research funds. From Dr. Marian Ropes, among others, came Boston's great training clinic in rheumatology. From all these forerunners who transformed arthritis during my wonder years rose my best chance to withstand it.

To perceive these processes then and today, a "miracle drug" is a promising mirror to look into. If I call the 1940s the "cortisone moment" for its sense of victory, fifty years later the moment and meaning have changed. Now we believe each cure gives rise to new symptoms, each victory releases threats. Everything good has side effects.

At our place in the Santa Cruz Mountains I see this paradox up close. We're clearing vines from old trees so they can grow—but who knew bare vines spill poison oak? In no time my rash runs so deep I want to scratch to the sinews. A home-care book commends hot showers for poison oak, so I take them. Cold oatmeal baths, says another. I lie limp in oatmeal and watch the rash spread subcutaneously, right through my cortisone-thinned skin. So this savage itching is worse because of a wonder drug. I take advice from John's aunt Ruth, who used cortisone for years against RA: "Thin, peelable, bruisable, altogether vulnerable skin—a consequence of steroid therapy—is not easy to live with, to be sure," she writes, "but the alternative is worse." Yes, RA is worse. After quitting cortisone, I shouldn't take more just for poison oak.

But mad with scratching, I sense my house is hiding leftover pills. One night I paw through shelves of soaps and cough drops, panting and feral until I find what I'm looking for. While John watches horrified, I stuff down a whole packet of steroids.

Oh, you world-class drug, I'll never go historical on you again. You're not a moment, you're a masterpiece. And the riddle of modern medicine rolls over and over me. What once made me better then made me worse. What then made me worse now makes me better. What now makes me better . . .

Better and worse, as anybody who has a chronic condition knows, can become a daily round-trip shuttle. In the mid-1990s, I find one thing that seems to move me on: remembering my life before the onset of RA. I go forward by getting back to the disease, by getting back *at* it. What I'm looking for is resistance stored up in the years before arthritis, a person prepared to turn with it, then against it.

The fifties prepared me to resist, without my knowing it. To recall that decade I ask the joints to let me look back through them. One day when I focus on painful fingers I see the outline of earlier ones. They're grasping my Esterbrook pen, all ink-stained with pages of fantasy, floating me from ninth-grade Pittsburgh toward London or Paris. This memory reveals how long I've been writing my way out of given conditions, and recalls something more. Around 1955 my dad confided that he imagined leaving Pittsburgh too, for a promised government job in Washington. But he'd belonged to a wartime circle—"a simple antifascist group, Mary"—later labeled Red. "Total falsehood," he said. "Washington just didn't want progressives like me." He never got security clearance for a civil job.

In the nineties, seven years after his death, I unearth my parents' papers, question my brother, and finally recall the bitterness in our household during the fifties—against Washington for suspecting my dad, against Pittsburgh for baiting leftists, against Communists for confounding his causes, against rising falsehoods.

Back then my mom used this bitterness like ammonia, for social cleansing. As personnel manager at Kaufmann's department store she placed "Negro" employees at the counters (to the customers' shock). Though she left this job to manage family personnel (following two million other postwar women who went home to be with the kids), she also practiced kitchen-table politics, gathering girlfriends to oppose segregation, to press the mayor for fair employment and "fairhousing" (as I heard the word), to serve the Child Guidance Center, and to raise money for Israel's new state. The mothers of my friends served me oven-made layer cake.

Alone in the kitchen after a fifth-grade day I was ready to trade my mother for the other kind until the thrilling moment when she rushed in and banged frozen Birds Eye peas and lamb chops into dinner. Her cooking made it clear the family was only one dish in her life. Of most mothers in fifties Pittsburgh, writer Annie Dillard recalls: "They coped. They sighed, they permitted themselves a remark or two, they lived essentially alone." But civic mothers left their *daughters* essentially alone, to become free-thinking busybodies from then on.

My first business was objecting to cosmetics and training bras, an entirely unpopular cause (and one that nudged me toward defending, in later years, women's right to have their bodies belong to themselves). I sneered at eighth-graders who crowded the bathroom checking bra straps, slicking on mascara.

"*You* will too," one told me.

"Bet I won't."

I barely touched makeup or bras for forty-five years to keep on winning that bet. Even back then I had another goal in mind: to run for student-body president. My campaign was managed by a son of Jonas Salk's, who came up with its slogan: "Have you SEEN her?" By the time the ballot came in, the president-elect knew how to run like a doll and win like a boy, and the trick stayed useful for years.

During that 1955 school year Pittsburgh kids were chosen as "polio pioneers," lining the school auditorium and proudly taking the shots, from Dr. Salk himself. Before puncturing my arm, he gently led me to a cot, noticing panic on my face, from shot-shyness but also from the idea that a disease could leave bodies permanently impaired. So far mine knew one bout of pneumonia, when my high fever came partly from fear that my friend Bobby would get it too and confess the lights-off game we called Five Minutes of Paradise.

Sickness and sex left only the faintest footprints in memory, until one day in '96 I empty an old box and find a 1955 diary kept locked for forty years:

Jan. 1. Dear diary, I'll be 14 in February. I have dishwater blond hair and blue eyes. I play the piano, and I'm crazy about boys.

Jan. 4. My brother wants to go to Harvard. Oh please, please God. I'd sacrifice anything if he could.

Jan. 10. Yesterday Mom gave up her volunteer job, and you know why? Because she didn't want to be away from home and me.

February 8. I've decided to make some vows: I will not speak sarcastically to my parents. I will not buy ice cream in school.

February 14. While a boy is kissing me I feel absolutely no emotion. But a day later, I have chills all day.

March 25. Jimmy told me I'm "too easy to neck with." I was always unsure about whether I was "fast" or not, but now I know.

March 27. P. told me in the elevator to hold a kiss longer. I proved I could for seven floors, but I won't French-kiss. I bluntly told him to "keep it American."

March 29. I'm trying very hard to lose weight even though I'm not fat.

April 9. Tonight I slept over at Lynn's. We soaped car windows, made taffy apples, smoked ourselves sick, and fried pickles in deep fat.

April 13. Dr. Salk just announced a cure for polio. God bless him. Polio is conquered! I feel so weirdly toward Jimmy.

May 4. Now I am truly happy! My brother got into Harvard. And I didn't sacrifice anything!

May 5. I am setting a *goal* for myself, the *Senior Award* for scholarship, leadership, and loyalty. It'll take me four years of work.

June 14. I want high grades on report cards so I'll have a good record. I want a good record so I can get into Radcliffe. I want to get into Radcliffe so I can make something of my life before I die off.

The eighth-grade girl of these green-inked pages, guarding her reputation, despising her "fat," holding her brother's future above her own, praising a mother who gives up volunteering, creating pleasure by retelling it—the girl who minded all the hedges of the fifties also trampled them, skeptical of her body's fate and awfully ambitious for her mind.

Apparently I was learning to balance output (good grades) against input (germs, calories, and tongues, for a start). By fourteen I'd been given to understand I might have a job someday but more to the point must stay slim. A job "because your husband might die," a prospect my dad etched fairly often. Slim because success seemed to be staked on my body. I remember my mom saying, "Don't count too much on work, because you'll give it up." Even volunteer work should be something to drop. After all, the average wife got married by twenty, just a few years away, and every woman I knew (except one aunt) was married with children and subsidized. You took care of your body so someone would take care of you.

In the teeth of this message I also planned to cure a major disease, like Dr. Salk.

In 1955, when our local genius became a national hero, announcing polio prevention, my parents rejoiced as if I'd be immune to any illness, now that our friend had created the vaccine in our hometown. Growing up among medicine men, and keeping my body safe, I was given to believe that I'd have whatever I hoped for. In Pittsburgh, where Dr. Salk, Dr. Spock, and Dr. Hench all started their work, the prestige of their research went unchallenged and carried over to other studies.

Forty years later, looking into medical history, I discover what some Pittsburgh medicine men had in store for my type of girl. A 1955 Pittsburgh study of "psychosocial factors associated with rheumatoid arthritis" warned of precisely the acts of ambition I was gearing up to commit. Reviewing fifty experiments, the study decided that RA sufferers had rejected the "female role" and shown "masculine protest reaction." Even their "physical activity is some sort of libidinous satisfaction, . . . a form of sublimation." Meanwhile men with RA endured something called "partial impotence." This "unsatisfactory sexual adjustment of rheumatoid arthritis patients" *fascinated* researchers, and I think I know why.

Stealing an idea here, an attitude there, they made arthritis stand for everything spooking the fifties: more moms at work when kids got home, more mental mess-ups. Without a solid link, they rushed to find "much in common" between "rheumatoid arthritis and schizophrenia." The root cause of RA that they ferreted out was—what else?—a "domineering, demanding mother." Did they fault my own mom, who trusted Dr. Spock's advice, surrendered her "masculine protest reaction" (a.k.a. her job), and stayed home to lay some Child Guidance on her kids? Was the side effect of research a new form of shame?

Looking back to the scare tactics used on women (you get out of line, you'll limp back in), I beam a standing ovation at the girl who worked toward class president and a senior award, because what would come at her from the fifties, as yet unknown, was the blame for a big disease.

As a teenager I had barely any notion of chronic illness, or how it was looked on, or that the middle-class fifties papered it over with the same creases and glosses they applied to race and sex. My teenage tendency, I recall, was to consider sickness a temporary state you're supposed to rise above.

And then in 1958, during the brief period of high school when I was not thinking how to be thinner, I decided to volunteer in a research hospital. Everything I saw there impressed me with the new curing power of medicine: I looked up to specialists and watched nurses take over patient care, learning it was less important. Likewise, chronic illness slipped behind an obscuring scrim that I only peered through later. At seventeen, working the reception desk, directing visitors to the urgent wards, I grew dimly aware that chronic patients went to crowded long-term facilities, elsewhere. When I delivered flowers, I imagined those dreadful wards as places where buds wouldn't stay fresh.

Thirty years later, rushing to my mother's room in the same hospital's gleaming wing for the well-insured, I took a wrong turn, went through a door, and found myself in 1958: a brown, non-air-conditioned corridor I'd never discovered back then, a long-term charity vault running side by side with the high-profile research wards.

Back then the medical-research drama captivated me, so I also volunteered in Jonas Salk's lab. After months there the head technician took me aside and whispered fiercely, woman to girl, "Don't you get stuck till you have a Ph.D."

"Stuck?"

"Women should have medical professions, not just medical problems."

"Oh." Professions, not problems. I filed that away.

At the time, I knew the National Foundation for Infantile Paralysis was supporting Dr. Salk's lab but not that it was heading from polio toward an "elusive search for the cause and cure of rheumatoid arthritis." By the late fifties that disease had finally gained research interest, diagnostic standards, antimalarial drugs, and a new journal called *Arthritis and Rheumatism*, but it stayed so "elusive" that one-third of women with RA, and one-fifth of men, never saw a doctor for their so-called aches and pains. Instead RA sufferers fantasized that "a dramatic cure" (as one of them said) "may suddenly be announced and that we will trek to schoolhouses throughout the land for immunizations." A Salk-minded society loved the polio plot, and so did I.

In fact I thought my medical village was about to cure the world—until I joined a high school program in Paris.

> July 5, '58. The women here are wearing their skirts almost
>   above their knees and gobs of makeup, to cover up their
>   sicknesses.
> July 26. On the train, French soldiers heading for Algeria put
>   their hands all over our necks and faces—a frightening
>   experience. My boyfriend Pierre says with rage, "C'est
>   une guerre sans fin."

It was the first time I saw someone my age defy a country's policies at all, let alone during a war, because some sicknesses, it seemed, could not be covered up. Before leaving France, I wrote:

> Aug. 4. We stopped at the Source Perrier, the biggest
>   racket ever invented. They take mineral water out of
>   the ground, add a little artificial flavoring and sell a very
>   small bottle of health.

> Aug. 25. I stopped in L'Humanité headquarters to get some
> Communist posters. The man there was quiet and beau-
> tiful and not the least rabble-rousing. He spoke of his
> cause like a religion.

What a reversal came about, that summer of '58. Imagine disputing a state at war, or using the high term *religion* to praise a Communist, or disparaging a fine corporate product as a "racket."

Coming home to my senior year, I suddenly relished my dad's outspoken ways. He walloped the kitchen table to approve Senator Estes Kefauver, who nailed drug companies for spending four times more on promotion than research, hoisting a $1.50 cost for my sick uncle's cortisone to $30 retail. Those price tags, said Kefauver, "under any standard are excessive," but what he proposed—licensing out medicines once the sales exceeded five times the cost—Congress just wouldn't pass.

Not then, not later, with drug companies pumping tens of millions of dollars into political campaigns, mostly Republican ones. In the nineties my pricey pill bottles prove there's no limit to pharmaceutical profit and power, and there's no money Americans won't throw at pain. In 1959 an Arthritis Foundation study, *The Arthritis Hoax*, showed consumers shelling out $250 million a year for fraudulent drugs and devices: Z-Ray applicators to stretch body atoms, costly tablets with one active ingredient (aspirin), $200 treatments in bankrupt uranium mines—remedies pushed by quacks in a battle against docs. *The Arthritis Hoax* scolded buyers for "wasting their money, . . . fritter[ing] away valuable time on quack preparations." Since wasting and frittering made the U.S. economy boom, these weren't fiscal sins but moral and female ones: the book's illustrations show foolish ladies holding up uranium mitts or basking under glow lamps. Meanwhile this first exposé of hoaxes "omitted" all treatments "prescribed by physicians" and all outsize company profits. Only the huckster and the housewife were on trial.

Why the housewife? I wonder. Then I remember Richard Nixon's key point in the 1959 "kitchen debate" with Soviet premier Nikita Khrushchev. Nixon claimed American products "make easier the life of our housewives." Even when he said this, I already doubted that American goods made Americans good. Or that hospitals took in all patients, or that all illnesses found vaccines, or that competition made companies fair and consumers aware.

But one primary falsehood pulled a fast one on me and the girls in my class of '59. We were positive that good grades and nice blond pageboys would open a full life for us. We went forth as seniors thinking prejudice couldn't apply to heads with hair like ours. There in the blast-furnace home of Iron City beer (pronounced "Arn-See," no need to add "beer") I belonged to the set that would drink Bloody Marys and leave town for college. Perched high above steelworkers, I simply didn't foresee the barriers ahead of well-schooled women.

My upbringing taught me to catch obvious hoaxes (pricey water and prescriptions, hyped-up cures and wars), but it took years of feminist history to show me deeper falsehoods left over from the fifties—not just the belief that ambition made females illness-prone but the notion that pivotal changes sprang from renowned sources. In fact unsung housewives like my mother brought social reform, and an unspoken disease like rheumatoid arthritis inspired a medical breakthrough.

At the end of the fifties my own breakthrough came when I carried off the senior award for "scholarship, leadership, and loyalty," the award I'd vowed to work for in my locked eighth-grade diary. At the high school awards ceremony the Latin teacher studied my face, as though peeling off my teenage dumb mask, and predicted, "The Ancients will assist you." I thought she was nuts, but in fact they do, decades later, when I learn their word *arthron*, for joint, which also refers to female genitals. In their view arthritis was caused in women by childbirth, or by "sorrow, care, and other passions of the mind."

Getting back into history, back into memory, begins bringing out the question of causes. Was my disease roused, as the ancients thought, by physical changes in childbirth? Or by passions of the mind?

About births and sorrows I ask the in-house professor of comedy: "Lie down with me, and tell any joke about this."

"OK," John starts. "A wife in labor cries out, '*Dieu! Quel douleur!*' The doctor holds back. This time she cries: '*Mein Gott! Die Schmerz!*' The doctor doesn't move. Then a third shriek: '*Oy vay! Oy vay!*' He says, 'Ah! Now it hurts.'"

"Oh great," I say. "The wife doesn't hurt till she gets down with Yiddish?"

"That's the point," John says. "Using high language—French or German—blocks real words for pain."

A silence falls, while I get down with real words: "Jesus, oy vay, it hurts."

John rolls over at once. "Oh no, love. What part?" He's asked this for years.

"Everywhere I have a joint."

By now, the mid-1990s, I know just how pain works on me and probably anyone who takes it chronic. My elbow brushes the mattress: enter the Jab. My fingers reach toward the night table: in comes the Zap. My shoulders register the Ache. My neck turns "tender" (a medical term of endearment) for the Torch. But at least these action figures sleep while I'm asleep. When their powers fade, my mind believes that nothing hurts, and my dreams feature agile limbs and warp-speed flying, with a tricky message: "I can do this!" My nerve system forgets it feels pain and even that it *needs* to forget.

Only now am I starting to grasp the waking mind's part in pain. In arthritis, medical sources say, pain starts when a swollen joint presses nerve endings and gets them firing. But when constant inflammation presses them over and over, they send nonstop signals to the brain. Then the brain lowers the nerves' threshold, causing a tinier stimulus to hurt even more. Pain from RA never diffuses like the scent of breakfast coffee. It gets stronger with time, a nasty twist. Anyone with RA has lots more trigger points firing at lower thresholds than anyone without. If I walk ten minutes too far, joints and muscles poke those points and actually *alter the nerves* to super-sensitive. They react when barely provoked, just from leaning on the mattress at night. Once-only injuries don't have time to rankle, but chronic inflammation deforms both joints and nerves, so that "minor changes of pressure," write researchers Ronald Melzack and Patrick Wall, "produce great surges of pain."

Until now I knew almost nothing about those surges, so I'm stunned to learn that "waves of chronic pain" (as described in David Morris's brilliant 1991 study) are "now sweeping over the modern world." To describe these waves, researchers formulate a revolutionary concept: pain arises from a complex "neuromodule," formed by injury *and* inflammation *and* moods *and* memories. To me this means that if I grab hold of memories, I might sometimes ride on top of pain.

At that thought I go to an attic box filled with papers from the sixties, when I first looked into mastering pain. In an old folder on natural childbirth I pick up the subject where I left off in 1968. Natural childbirth made use of a theory called "gate-control" by Melzack and Wall, a "genuine scientific revolution" of the sixties that gave rise to a thousand U.S. pain clinics. Gate-control posits that nerve fibers carry messages to and *from* the mind, transmitting sensory signals and emotional ones too. If a pain stimulus "exceeds a critical level," the brain can redirect or close the route. It can even be trained to do this. In Reynolds Price's *A Whole New Life* "the secret of living with pain is wanting hard to throw it out of central control." That's what natural childbirth would do for labor pain, I thought—not knowing labor would be just the opening thwack.

I remember telling John in '68 that childbirth would go fine because I was "boning up on pain!"

"Good. Down you go." He pointed to the floor, where we had our nightly natural-childbirth practice. "Ankle ready?"

"Ready," I nodded, knowing he'd pinch my Achilles tendon to simulate the sharpness of birth pangs while I breathed deep and distracted my mind. What my mind registered anyway: how hard it is to take pain, even for practice. I only hoped labor worked like grad school, and I'd pass because I'd cram.

"It used to be worse," I ventured, "when Descartes described pain as a long bell rope in the body ringing in the steeple." John squeezed for Descartes, and I rolled away. The brain as a belfry, having its rope jerked, offended my free will in 1968, whereas gate-control made pain my own mental job. When John pressed the tendon harder, I reminded myself that pain is just "a communication," as sociologist Thomas Szasz wrote at the time, allowing me to yell, "You're hurting my heel," and take charge of it. A little gate-control was the armor I'd use in childbirth, pretending John was squeezing my Achilles tendon till the baby came out. How lucky for me that pain got explained as perception of pain, just when I was practicing for it.

Decades later I notice the sting in sixties research on pain. As the idea spread that mental outlooks can reduce pain, researchers latched onto pain resistance as a measure of worth, for individuals and for ethnic groups. They designed studies implying that noble sufferers like African Americans were inherently braver than others, such as Jews, who always "complained loudly." Reading these studies in the nineties, I'm sighing, "Spare me," for they made outspoken anxiety an inborn Jewish trait, just years after the Nazis. When Jewish women yelped louder than Protestants as a pressure cuff squeezed their arms, sixties researchers concluded that "ethnic membership (e.g., Italians, Jews)" induced an "exaggerated expression of pain." Does "exaggerated" sound a tad prejudicial? A famous 1969 study, People in Pain, depicted Jews questioning doctors while a Yankee stayed detached "like a good American." Guess which group was viewed by the medical staff (without direct measures of pain) as "deviants, hypochondriacs, and neurotic"? Likewise, a prestigious 1968 study highlighted women's "more subjective symptoms" and the "excess chronic illness reported by women as compared with men." Are "more subjective" and "excess" neutral? When researchers clucked at Jewish mothers for reading a "slight sensation of pain . . . as a sign of illness," when they honored Yankees for telling a child to take it "like a man," when they examined arthritis and with pretty thin data fixed on a "difference in the pain response due to ethnocultural factors," was every non-Yankee non-male sentenced for fussing too much?

I rest my face on the library table. All the sixties scrutiny of chin-up Yankees, noisy Jews, stoic Negroes, excessive women would be dropped in a dustbin instead of cited for decades—except for that brand-new theory: the brain makes the pain.

I can't help wondering if medicine at the time—that is, at the time pain and disease came to me—decided even RA was caused by the mind. Did psychic flaws (which I was apparently subject to) become as much a part of arthritis research as brilliant breakthroughs?

On a scorching day, when it's a joy to sit in air-conditioned stacks reading articles on agony, I sift through 1960s studies, finding one called "Personality Factors Associated with Rheumatoid Arthritis" that targets traits like "perfectionist" or "self-sacrificing." Physicians singled out a disturbed personality as "one of the necessary conditions for the genesis" of RA. They asserted RA's "psychosomatic aspects." Sometimes they degraded it to a "psychosomatic disorder." A sixties account by an RA-suffering journalist well-aware of medical theories pegged away at her own faults: "So often, so very often, does a period of unusual anxiety and strain correspond with the onset or rapid advance of the disease." Here in the medical shelving I finally see what that decade had me believing: that by becoming, like many women in those years, a "perfectionist" susceptible to stress, I grew prone, in my inmost nature, to a shame-laden disease.

I ask myself again whether I learned, long ago, to imagine RA roused by passions of the mind.

Stress, 1997

Even today the "psychosomatic" slant in sixties studies skews health books. Many of them claim you make yourself healthy and imply you most likely made yourself ill.

For a valid test of whether mental stress made me ill, I'm waiting on results from the National Databank for Rheumatic Diseases, which is looking into this question, gathering psychological data from a widespread questionnaire to be filled out twice a year. The trouble is, the Databank isn't getting simple answers, not from me:

How much of the time have you felt calm and peaceful?

I used to check "Most of the time" to ace the test. Now I'm tempted to answer, "Calm with RA? You're kidding." Should I feel "peaceful" when I don't know, for instance, if my children might inherit my disease?

Secretly I don't believe the Angel of Anatomy would pass it on. No one seems to have passed it to *me*, after all. But looking into it, I find mixed news about RA transfer. (My folder on genetics, opened without good-grip hands, litters the floor and adds to the biblical Sea of Reeds where Alek practices clarinet.) Genes called HLA-DR, special immune particles that tell self from nonself, may make RA more likely and more severe. Still, most people with the gene don't break out with the disease. Native Americans have the highest incidence of RA, and Mexican Americans are quite susceptible, while African Americans and Asians aren't: these facts point suspiciously to genetic influences, though RA passes much less clearly from parent to child than other autoimmune diseases do. That's about as far as researchers go, which I can live with.

But where's the calm in knowing that another partially genetic disease, Alzheimer's, left my mother utterly dependent, and a stroke made my father ask to live with his kids? May my joints rot in hell if they ever make me ask this of mine.

"Calm and peaceful"?

I check off, "Not much of the time."

In the last six months how often did you feel as if nothing turned out the way you wanted it to?

For years I've given nice answers to cheer up the Databank. Well, this time I'm letting it rip. Nothing turned out the way I wanted it to. My musings about RA are filling the recycle bin, my genocide course keeps adding manmade curriculum, and my joints hurt no matter what I feel about life.

Agree or Disagree: It seems as though fate and other factors beyond my control affect my condition.

I ought to "disagree." Researchers think moping about fate and feeling powerless may actually make arthritis worse. But I have to scrawl "Agree." You bet. "Of *course* fate controls my condition, or I'd blow it off."

Agree or Disagree: No matter what I do, or how hard I try, I just can't seem to get relief.

Agree *and* disagree. It's a trick question. On one side a tantrum in the joints won't "get relief." On the other "tantrum" sounds easier than "endless burning." Some people try for relief by wedging a metaphor into illness. Anatole Broyard saw cancer as "an affair with a demented woman." After a mastectomy Audre Lorde envisioned "the Amazons of Dahomey," African warriors with cut-off breasts. Arthur Frank found illness metaphors "a kind of retrospective necessity."

On the way to a metaphor of my own I look at Emily Dickinson, who felt "Zero at the bone," but I could use a less chilling image. Turning to the Song of Songs, the Biblical poem touching on body parts, I find "the joints of thy thighs are like jewels." A bit rosy? Instead I try an honorable old phrase: "a man of parts," an aggregator of properties. A *woman of parts*—there's my metaphor. A woman of parts stores her scraps inside a pantry of skin, but with so many fragments it's not possible for her to survive without help. To keep the parts in one estate, she has to have connections, and she has to have supports.

This woman of parts completes the Databank questionnaire and carries her parts to consult a rheumatologist at Stanford Medical Center.

Since the examining room is quiet, I start making up my own questions. If asked how my disease is progressing, I'll admit I've been losing joints, hair, voice, trust. Questioned further I'll say I've made lots of small moves in the last years. I've absorbed cortisone and methotrexate, nudged the state for assistance, tracked my old disease into modern forms, kept a private account of RA, and searched the public shelves for other ones. If pressed I'll mention turning to my own past, tracking my first decades and the ways they set me up for arthritis. I'll even reveal my best move—refocusing the mind from a malady to the story of a malady.

When the researcher finally walks in, he asks right off the bat, "The medications you've been on so far?" That's all.

"Methotrexate, gold, antimalarials, prednisone, aspirin, ibuprofen, you name it."

"Methotrexate: how long?"

"Four years or so."

"Gold and steroids?"

"Cortisone, maybe three years? Probably more. The gold injections went on for—some time." And I draw salary for being a historian.

He tries another tack. "How would you rate, on a scale of one to ten, your condition right now?"

"An eight? No, I guess it's been worse. A five?"

It's unnerving to see my disease in unconnected dots. On the examining table I figure out what I have to do: create a decent case history, a regular report of goings-on inside my joints.

For my next checkup I prepare a nicely typed page with all my drugs, activities, questions:

> GENERAL HEALTH: Feeling tired. Teaching less than full-time.
>
> JOINTS: Left arm losing mobility. Right ankle swollen and collapsing.

Writing these phrases astonishes me. They draw most of my fear to the surface the way a scalding shower sucks itching to the skin. Before each doctor's visit from then on I design a full report that faults my body joint by joint but at the same time declares me a going concern, all long-term losses and short-term gains accounted for. I become the independent auditor of my own (mid-risk) corp.

My doctor (I note with quiet pleasure) slips my quarterly reports right into the medical record, as if instructed by *The Illness Narratives*, where Arthur Kleinman favors patients asking, "What is the cause of the disorder?" and "What is the source of improvements and exacerbations?" I don't want to imagine what caused the disorder, but I would like to say how it's grown. I'd like a chart showing how each common stage prompts a personal response.

STAGE	RESPONSE
Onset: I first felt ill.	**Disbelief:** "You mean *me?*"
Diagnosis: I started treatments.	**Depression:** "Can't go through this."
Remedy: I applied aggressive drugs.	**Readiness:** "I'll try anything."
Remission: My symptoms ran out.	**Amazement:** "What did I do right?"
Recurrence: My malady turned worse.	**Despondency:** "How'd I go wrong?"
Advance: The damage turned irreparable.	**Resistance:** "I'd make a fist if I could make a fist."

Laying out these stages, I wonder how my doctors narrated them. Dr. B. continues the rare practice of dictating notes in my presence, but I want to read my entire medical record, now that patients have that right. Equipped with doctors' views and my own I can take Kleinman's advice: build "an illness narrative that will make sense of and give value to the experience."

On request, a staff person at my clinic dredges up four bulging folders, 1960s through 1990s, and sits two feet away, making sure I don't rip off pages or weep all over the bone scans. In fact it's a hoot: I've been wriggling out of operations and shrugging off medicines for years. A close look reveals not just tons of lab work but a real-life plot. Here's an unsuspecting woman who gets sick, stays sick, takes things hard; her body changes, the culture changes, new treatments check in. The touching fact is that my doctor records all this—what I look like, how my family gets along, where my work takes me, whether my bones move.

The term *medical record* doesn't begin to cover the enterprise. It reveals this woman of parts as more than the sum of them. It comprises the only biography, slanted of course and biochemical, ever made of me.

Nothing less than a chronic disease has ever inspired such a record or given value to my seasons of trouble, moments of forgetting, hours so involved in family or films that the mind detached from the body, or hours when nothing could spring it free.

Because of reaching back into the past, I'm readier now to imagine what else I can do with RA, to give something new a shot.

IV. Getting Help

> Though you may call it love,
> doctors call it rheumatism

Cole Porter

> Rheumatism is any pain occurring
> within a mile of a joint.

Philip Hench

Family, 1997

"Wanna fly?" Alek calls to me one afternoon, keen to lift a sport kite into a Pacific headwind.

My hands wince.

"Wanna fly?" my teenager calls again.

"Sure," my fingers wave, though these days they aren't up to tugging a lamp cord, let alone a six-foot sport kite hauled to a hilltop near home. Alek bounds over, wraps handkerchiefs around my wrists, stands behind with his arms circling me, cups his knuckles over mine, and squeezes the strings between his fingers. When our arms snap back, I pitch against him, but he does the pulling, the kite rips skyward, and our little tugs widen in the air to huge arabesques. Down here my feet hold the ground like pickets, but I'm up there too, zipping across the sun.

At that instant I decide it's worth any stretch, short of gluing a kite and a kid on each arm, to get a liftoff like this again. Whatever it takes, I'm going to kick against the gravity in my life.

A minute later, with the kite bouncing on the grass and my wrists unhooked, I stand stock-still. Even lifting my arms a few minutes has caused more pain than I know what to do with.

"You OK?" asks Alek.

"Don't you worry," I tell him, meaning I know you do worry.

Eyes pinched shut, I realize it took a whole family to lift the wingspread just now. Sarah taught her brother how to launch this kite, her boyfriend Scobie designed it, John snapped a picture of it, Alek found a way to rig me up, and I got a one-time shot at taking wing. A whole collective helped me off the ground.

From that moment my reluctant joints seem to do more than drag my attention down, as they used to. They still act as separators—that's

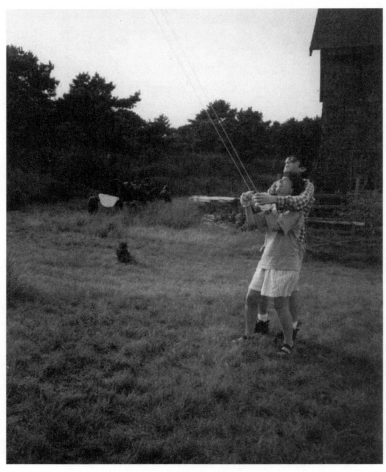

Kite-flying, 1997. Photo by John Felstiner.

real. But now they can link me to the people I belong with. In a string
of occasions they'll become my main connectors.

So some months later, expecting my joints to serve me at family
events, I'm heard mumbling "Nothing to wear."

"At Sarah's wedding?" John asks.

"I mean, what *can* I wear? With running shoes." As usual my ankle
has seized and my foot bone lowered, and if you've seen a piano with its
keys sprung, you've seen my toes. I can't imagine any new dress going

with my double-width trainers, so I make it my business not to get one. "It's bad to look odd," I moan to John, "when I want all eyes on Scobie and Sarah."

"You'll look fine."

Will I? A whole year ago the date was set, and still the mother of the bride is missing an outfit, waiting for news from her feet.

Finally my sister-in-law Susan comes over to help me choose clothes. She gets me out of carrier-class shoes and into rubber sandals, the kind I leave the shower with.

The next morning, down a grassy aisle at Stanford, Sarah walks gracefully between John and me, gently holding one of us steady until we deliver her to Scobie. They play an Irish duet on flute and pennywhistle, marry each other in English and Hebrew, and dash off, feet flying, for an hour alone. When everyone gathers for dinner, the joy on Sarah's face as she toasts Scobie, and on Scobie's as he plays saxophone for her, and on Alek's as he hugs his sister, lifts my heels. Lightly I slow-dance with John but sit out the fast ones, knowing my limits. Then I come back and hear someone call, "Mary rocks!" as rhythm grabs the feet, sways the hips, takes me by surprise. To boogie at Sarah's wedding: who would have hoped for that?

A week later my shame over shoes seems senseless. Why should decorum matter on my feet? Sinking into my armchair, I try to think back through the joints, back to 1900 when my four grandparents made it to America and their feet were their fortune. Lamed or maimed they wouldn't survive. They had to stand on the deck, stand before officials, stand in line, stand behind the counter, stand in line some more, stand at the stove, stand on the sidewalk to peddle, stand to teach Hebrew, stand to wring laundry, stand to say prayers in shul, stand to wash dishes after Shabbos. Their children would never forget their standing in this country. Later my dad favored genteel footwear in hopes of becoming someone who might, on occasion, just sit down—say, at a Fourth of July picnic or a university table. His buffed shoes and sturdy garters (which even hosiery salesmen couldn't identify now) were matched by my mom's fine hose, in which she walked smartly out of a shabby immigrant neighborhood. But why she hoarded a hundred pair I can't imagine till I recall her post-Depression fear of being "down at the heel." Hosiery is the only clothing of hers I've saved, each pair rolled and at the ready in a dresser. Nylons in waiting swell upward every time Alek or Sarah yanks open the Memorial Stocking Drawer for me.

With this legacy I actually step through arthritis expecting to stay in stride. So whenever my lowest joints refuse their job and undermine my base, it's an affront to the walks of life my parents and grandparents passed on to me. I know they kept their footing, and I should do the same.

But I also learn from my present family to trust in change. The hose-and-garter generation couldn't have imagined my sandals or my children's flip-flops. Even John and I are startled, when we visit Alek's music camp, to find him performing quartets, quintets, octets, bare-foot. For five weeks he puts shoes away, stumbles over roots, pounds along gravel, lets his soles get filthy and scratched. It's the sign of a third-generation American to be that foolhardy with feet.

Since flying the kite with Alek, I've felt buoyed by the generations around me. When Sarah and Scobie visit us from Seattle (where she teaches preschool and he designs high-performance kites), this sense of lift comes again. At a play-along *Messiah* in Stanford Church the updraft of Sarah's flute and a deep bubbling from Alek's clarinet and a "Hallelujah" from my own voice swish around the cupola—an ascension if I ever heard one. That night I dream of rising in the air.

The next morning John says, "So when you dream—I never asked you this—your feet don't hurt?"

"We-ll, no."

"Good! You haven't let arthritis in."

That *is* good, I think, clapping my palms on my temples.

Another morning I see John smile in his sleep before it's quite seven. No wake-up sounds, since Alek left yesterday for a youth orchestra tour. I listen for a thunk (seventeen-year-old body flung from bed), a phtt (icebox opened), a pop (cartons on the counter), a thud (backpack dropped at the door), a boom-bap (radio hip-hop). The house is quiet, a preview of all the years he won't be in it.

"God, I miss the decibel energy of him," I say, and just then his vacant room fills with wild noise from his preset radio. I leave it be.

The next day at seven the radio breaks into my dream of flying, as if what's drifting away (a son here, a joint there) is still around.

By Sunday Alek is back home to turn off his alarm, but I wake early anyway, eager to take him to San Francisco's science museum for the afternoon. Wandering through it, we somehow enter the evolution exhibit at the wrong end. In our direction lizards turn into dinosaurs, birds into fish, humans into apes. Forwards, evolution seems fairly proverbial. Backwards, I'm thunderstruck by the causal links, how our expanded brains grew from an upright stance, which grew from— what? A new improved hip joint, strongly seated to move our legs forward, while gorillas jiggle at the hips like skeletons on the Day of the Dead. I turn back through evolution just to be sure. Yes. From a hip we rose to a stance, to a brain, then to a human being. Joints started all that.

I ascend a nearby staircase, moving slowly but with all the stability of my species, and turn at the top, proud sapiens, to give the joints a bow.

The next morning I read in poet Louise Bogan's journal, "Long continued pain reduces one to the state of a blustering child." So I tell my family, "I'm not a blustering child. I don't *always* need help," as I limp across the kitchen. Alek, our democrat at the breakfast table, takes me down a peg. "You expect to be Bravejoint?"

Yes, I do. I've had a word with the Angel of Anatomy. So long as I act brave, no disasters, in all fairness, should happen to us.

But one night storm waters ooze through our concrete foundation, the sump pump inhales and exhales like an iron lung, and then the power goes out. In darkness the water rises. "What we need is a bailing brigade," I say, and the family falls into cast: John the captain, Alek the do-it-all bosun, myself the first mate. "You two carry pails and dump the water outside. I'll do the door." Bravejoint can't make it alone.

By one a.m. John is wincing and Alek's carrying both buckets, but the water rises higher. "I'm calling this," I say. "You'll break your backs."

For two more days the seepings undermine our walls and shift the family seat.

"At least we're safe," says John.

"Time being," is all I say.

"It's just this once."

I know better.

I know chronic. I sniff it all day, being someone who can't keep her footing like her forebears, or wear proper shoes to a wedding, or carry buckets in a crisis. But hold on: the point is to pass the test of time, like evolutionary joints. With this in mind I leave the mud-based house behind and head to a concert with John and Alek.

At first I swear they ought to have me ditched. It takes so long to push my arms through a coat, get the damn thing zipped, open the car door, spoon me in, buckle my seatbelt, press the lock, that before we get going, we're already late, and guess who's to blame. What I do when we pull into a full parking lot is look around for reprieve: a front-line place to match my blue disabled-driver placard, next to the sign saying that without that plastic we owe $295 to the state. Now the family animation runs in reverse: open Mary's door, unsnap her seatbelt, yank her by the armpits, hobble her to the entryway.

I turn to my nearest and dearest and say, "You gotta stick with me, folks. I'm your parking space."

Partners, 1998

"It's just a drag on my family," I tell a visiting friend, "my *always* having RA."

"But you get help from them."

"Of course. More than help."

"From John?"

"Most of all from John."

Since it's a sunny day and I feel pretty good, we browse San Francisco until my RA and my friend's chronic fatigue deposit us on a bench. "No one really gets it, do they?" I say.

"Not this bit-by-bit collapse."

A few days later her voice on the phone sounds choked as her story comes out. When she arrived home, her husband of many years was waiting at the door, but the suitcase he took in hand wasn't hers. It was his. He was leaving, he announced. Moving out. Apparently he'd braved her first fatigues but couldn't face the chronic part. After a minute she adds, "Husbands want their wives back."

Their lives back, I'm thinking. They contract for better or for worse, not for worse and worse. I shiver for myself too. Not frightened—terrified. *Anyone* might leave because a partner's illness turns too intense or boring or lasts too long. It takes months before my friend's husband and his suitcase walk back in, dripping with remorse. It takes months before I ask John, "What'll we do when I get worse?"

"We'll manage."

Or will he shear off again, now that I no longer have two working arms to put around him? Now that my hips have problems besides how I think they look from behind? Suddenly I hear a click, a snapping together of private and common doubts. Surely I'm not the only disjointed woman unsure of her appeal.

At night I read aloud a clipping lifted from my doctor's waiting room. A woman with RA writes, "On bad days, you just can't have any kind of intimate relationship, sexual or otherwise."

"Let's skip otherwise," John says, and we turn to each other, though not so easily as we lie together apart.

The next night I read another true story. A woman in a wheelchair hears someone exclaim, "You must be a saint." This is said to the husband wheeling her along. I tell John, "Pushing a stroller, a man's a dad. Pushing a wheelchair, he's a saint." As John's hand tucks under my armpit to help me walk, I whisper, "You're opening your wings."

"Mostly your milk cartons."

"Good God, what expertise. Do you wonder," I ask him, "how a woman with arthritis still gets furious at you?"

"For what?"

For your advantages, your speed, your liberty, your once-a-year checkups, your tappa-tappa keyboard, your finished drafts, your arm muscles, your—"For being the one nearby. For striding around with those powers able-bodied men have," which are powers I'm afraid I love. "And for being more equal than me."

"Why let it bother you?" he asks. "Why not stay equal to your tasks each day?"

"Because I'm not the one who gets to not be sick."

Later John bends into a stretch, then jogs uphill while I slouch in a chair. As soon as he gets home, I let a crazy furor loose. I've just noticed my tape recorder malfunctioning, chewing up three weeks of work. John's comforting: "There's a good chance you'll be able to retrieve this." My reaction is cool: I'll throw away three weeks of his writing, then say precisely what he said to me: "There's a good chance . . ." Just a fantasy. I'll Xerox it first.

If I need to lighten resentment, he needs to concede the trickiness of health, for he loses sight of his frailties and feels too strong by comparison. One day at our place in the mountains I see him roll a stump up the path to make a seat of it, risking a back spasm that could put him prone for days.

"You're crazy," I say. "But let's go sit there. Oh! It's wonderful," and my knees give in to it. Then I bobble on my swollen right ankle till John jacks me up the hill, hoisting my underarm like a British bobby: "Come along with me, Miss."

In the cabin he suddenly slaps his lower spine. "Not now," I cry out. Not a spasm now, when there's no one who can lift him. But as he whips off his shirt, I see a tick corkscrewing in. The tweezers that my no-account fingers drop are caught by him in midair, and he twists them counterclockwise to extract the tick behind his back. It's easy to believe he *deserves* his able body when he's so fine in a pinch.

The plain truth is, it takes more than John's handiness to keep us going. It takes two paychecks and double health plans, making me wonder how people survive without our safety net. Probably by chain reaction, like the song where a woman swallows a fly and then gulps a spider to deal with the fly, and on from there.

> Says a woman with RA: I can't get out of bed today.
> Says her boss along the way: You stop work you get no pay.
> Says her partner in dismay: Find a cheaper place to stay?
> Says the woman with RA: Cheaper place is cold all day.
> Says RA: Got you, eh?

Knowing these binds, I can't manage to sound upbeat in a talk I call "When One of Us Is Ill." I start by quoting researchers' triple negatives (the closest they get to positive): "One cannot rule out, by insisting on the negative character of illness and its effect, that some forms of 'secondary gain' are not possible." Gain from illness? I'm impatient with anyone's belief in this.

"Don't you discover strengths in yourself when ill?" asks a listener.

Strengths you'd trade in a heartbeat for health.

"Don't spouses give each other care?"

Women give more time. Men spend more change.

"But women get support from partners."

Yes, but you'd best be born male before getting ill.

"Then where does love come in?"

Time-out for that one.

A week later the answer comes when I hear my friend Estelle praise her partner for the way she handles diminished sight: "What attracted me in the first place was her taking a limit as a challenge."

"You love her for carrying the loss?"

"Yes," Estelle says.

"You mean if Julia Roberts played a Pretty Woman whose eyes go bad and hips need operations, you'd love her for coping with changes?"

"Yes, Mary."

At that instant I know where love comes in. Love is what you take and give *with* someone's inability, not in spite of it.

Suddenly today's anger is cooler than yesterday's. Rather than rage at the flesh of my flesh, it's a matter of weighing our lives on different scales. To give up being equal with John, always a scuffle at best, I envision separate tracks in this event. What keeps us parallel: We both draw on stores of fear, we top up with compassion, and we're good for some laughs.

For the moment John is spry but doesn't know for how long.

Here the edge is mine. I already live with what he fears.

His desire: to go on able as he is. Mine: to grow weaker with a tab of dignity.

His ambition: to keep active. Mine: to stay zesty.

His hope: the same as mine—when one of us is ill, two will take the heat.

The next morning: "John. Feel my arm, the upper part. Chilly, right? Now feel the elbow joint."

"OW-W-W," he shouts, alarmed after all these years that something so steamy lives in a temperate frame.

My faith is in that shout. When he leans over and kisses the outer corner of my elbow, I think, Oh yes, it's all right, I'll get started on this day.

Time, 1998

My day starts with flicking on a miked phone, a speech-enhanced computer, an electric letter opener, and a power stapler. John's workday supports historic preservation, with a rotary phone, a pre-Windows computer, a wooden pencil. My day looks for fresh means of self-help. To release my family I dream of joint-saving gadgets like push-button fridge doors or pedal-operated jar openers and hope I'll find them by subscribing to *Electronic House*.

That hope just might be misplaced. *Electronic House* sees my kitchen as a situation room, with my dishwasher sending code in Quiet Scrub and my appliances snooping on my children. It drives home the fact that everything I touch is timeworn. My stove, at the pulsing heart of Silicon Valley, doesn't self-light or self-clean, though it does match the one-cycle washer. As my fantasy of progress fades, I dial the rotary and cancel my subscription. The automated voice says, "Please press one."

Ah, time-saving electronics. That's where you'll really get help, everyone says. But the more people live at chip speed, the more people like me fall behind. "It's hard being in touch with you," say my friends, now that e-mail is everyone's handshake. Without working hands "I *receive* e-mail," I apologize, "but I don't give." Sadly, revolutions discard their losers: artisans, natives, homebodies, and now the digitally off-line.

Guest lecturing in a Stanford history class, I mention all this and am amazed at how many healthy-looking students tell me afterward their overstressed hands can't work the mouse. Face it: that's historical slippage. One student, however, suggests Dragon NatSpeak, a newly designed speech-recognition program priced to compete with IBM. That day the *New York Times* says speech programs are "changing the way many people interact with computer chips." Interacting with computer chips may fall a snippet short of my goal, but I do like the means of advancement here. Switching on my tape recorder, I exhale a few sentences: "Just as the Jacuzzi was invented by a father helping his joint-crippled son, just as aspirin came from a son helping his rheumatoid father, just as universal design—automatic doors, touch screens, wheelchair curbs—make everyone proficient, now disabled needs break into speech technology. The so-called losers shoot us forward."

In this spirit I'm after ways to use digital speech without destroying my voice. I'm consulting IBM, going inside with Intel, joining the techies above the keyboard tappers. For once I'm the future, Electronic Woman, Princess of Power, Pentium Chip.

In practice, though, I'm never caught speeding with speech recognition. One lecture for my biography course takes eight hours to produce, owing to the program's resistance to my ideas. Exasperated, I offer one last sentence for it to pulverize: "Thelonious Monk died of a cerebral aneurysm, but his reputation was renewed by Wynton Marsalis." The program is flawless on Thelonious Monk, Wynton Marsalis, and "cerebral aneurysm," which I can't spell myself. It misses "died of" and "but his" and "by."

"Quick!" I yell for Alek. "My computer knows Thelonious. Tell me other composers you like." Then I repeat each name, eyes closed: "Alek likes Sergei Prokofiev. Alek likes Dmitri Shostakovich, John Coltrane, Giuseppe Monteverdi, Gustav Mahler, Hildegard von Bingen." I open up. Perfect score: no flies on this database. It does, however, dislike "Alek likes." How intriguing that my software imitates my soft tissues, giving respect to major organs and blowing off the crucial little connectors.

Trying a lecture for my genocide course, I discover the program's partisan and prurient mind. It refuses to recognize "Nazi." I mean, it refuses the word and also explains: "not see, not see."

"You damn well better see," I shout, finger cocked over the power button. "Fine. I'll pluralize."

I say, "Nazis." It writes, "Not seize," as if I'm Chamberlain at Munich.

I see "mountains of evil in the Nazi era." It says they're "Not Sierra."

I go cell by cell. It goes: sell buy sell.

I divide body from soul. It devises body from Seoul.
I plug mikes into jacks. It plugs Mike's into Jack's.
I like circadian rhythms. It likes Sir Katie and Rhythms.
I walk off the trail. It walks off betrayal.
I point toward denial. It points toward the Nile.
I hint delights. It hits the lights.
I look for dauntless speech. It looks for topless beach.

"Speech recognition works best with my eyes closed," says a poet in the student cafeteria, where we're discussing her brain injury and my elbows.

I'm humbled. "What draws you to writing poetry then?"

"The short lines. Now can I ask you how RA affects what *you* write?"

"I can't do a thing to make words come out fast."

Faster, damn you! I always order, then hear the desperation in my voice. I'm going to have to get time on my side, along the lines of Barbara Hillyer's *Feminism and Disability*: "It doesn't matter how long it takes you. It's not a race. It's your life and you can choose the pace." Choosing the pace—an hour to make my computer write a letter, a good minute to take off a sock—I tell my friends Mary and Emily, "Go on ahead, I'm slow," but they say, "There isn't one right speed. What matters is the effort." I assume they mean with the sock.

People I like a lot, usually, take for granted their turnaround deadlines or quickie lectures written on planes. Even my family shifts the noun *time* into a hyperactive verb. John clocks himself as a runner, Alek praises a wind quintet that performs "tight," Sarah talks of hustling for the Russian judge.

"What's a Russian judge?"

"When an Olympic athlete gets scores like 9.9, 9.9, and 5.9, that's the Russian judge."

"Oh, honey. Only a true 9.9 would think of that." And she's right. Even a split-second delay means not good enough.

At night I read that disabled people "provide special insight into the nature of time in our society." Mornings I do my best to provide special insight to commuters on a local train. Many days I scuttle from my connecting bus to the train at top speed (for me) only to watch the steel doors close. To the insiders I'm the person who could make hundreds of them late. Out here in the cold it's one measly minute. Waiting for the next train, I invent a workday set by clocks with gnarled hands, with hours graduated by need, and one Minute of Downtime for compassion.

Compassion, the force that stretches time, counts all day long. In the morning a sweater that buttons up the front arrives from my friend Zaza, who knows I can't top-load my clothes. At a noon lecture I start to wiggle out of it, and my friend Marilyn reaches over two seats to pull it from my shoulders. On the way out my ankle buckles, and my friend Betsy has to grab my arm. OK, I'm labor-intensive. But friends keep recapturing time for me.

And I devote more time to them as my body loses its gait. Every February I renew friendships in a workshop of feminist history teachers. Every March a few college chums fly across the country for days of unhurried walks and talks. Twice a year my intimates, Emily and Mary, travel with me, watch my energy, and tell me, "Take it nice and slow." Every month my writers' group assures me I'm moving along just fine. Every week Ruth and I have an eight o'clock phone call, taking time for affection.

One night on the phone Ruth says once again, "After cancer what's there to be afraid of?" and we remember there's never an *after* arthritis, a release from slowness or loss. I live in a body that insists on its presence, all the time.

"If you get help from friends," says my older friend Hannah on our once-a-year outing to the San Francisco Botanical Garden, "in time you'll pass it to another person." We stroll through ferns unfolding from fiddles, dropping leaves, renewing. If only my joints could grow fresh like that.

"I can't see the point of a body signaling pain time after time."

"It's a message to change," Hannah says.

"And if changing doesn't help?"

"Then try something else."

"And if nothing works?"

"Think about living less long."

"Oh." As we stroll away, Hannah adds, "You prepare yourself for less time by giving care. Then others will care for you."

"I get that lesson already from arthritis—to be a friend to friends."

"Good, because pain can distort your view, make you think the world centers on you, make you hard on people close by." My wise friend stops beside an ancient fern, both of them giving shade to newer sprouts, passing time along.

I walk in silence, thinking that I don't whine to friends about pain and hardly mention it to my children, trying to save them from sadness or pity or fear, but to John—to John I pile it on. Somehow he absorbs my complaints. Somehow we go on mending and remaking our marriage. At that thought my heart lurches a little.

If pain is a message to change, as Hannah said, it's to change what I *see* (I can't change what I feel) in the joints. From architect Louis Kahn I'm taking an idea of the joint as the beginning of ornament. Does this mean design requires junctions, just the way history needs human meetings? "No joints, no history," I tell John one night in the car.

We're en route to a performance by choreographer Merce Cunningham, whose program surprises us by calling joints "independent entities that can move . . . as if each movable body part had a mind of its own." Cunningham later comes onstage, knees bowed with arthritis, hips oaken. He grimaces. I hold my breath. Then he grins. Suddenly I grasp the sense of time I've been looking for: stiffened but still spirited, still moving.

The time my friends and I give each other affirms our desire to help. Sometimes acquaintances offer help too, asking if I've tried a favored herb or massage, and usually I mean to, sometime. Have you tried psychotherapy? they ask. Of course. For anyone with a chronic illness I consider it a human right (though insurance excludes it from the package). My sharp and kindly therapist does what no other medical helper can: she refuses to leave me comfortless.

Have you tried acupuncture? Of course. I've tried a Chinese-trained doctor who said acupuncture works partly "by placebo," by symbolic means, and swore he had the chops to cure me. Not so. Then I tried an M.D. who admitted, "Acupuncture has a hard time with rheumatoid arthritis." I gave it another six months but still couldn't swivel to pull out the car afterward. Now I'm trying a practitioner who wants to "tonify my yin," and I keep coming just to hear that phrase. Her acupuncture needles thrill me with Qi, Chinese circuitry inside the skeleton. She also hands me French clay to make a poultice, a prescription in Mandarin for herbs, and an African nut butter unknown to my neighbors. She hopes my body turns "pukka—you know that word? In India it means ripe." I've got a whole world order pulling for me. Though none of this turns out to touch RA, it makes me feel pukka, and that's good enough for now.

Now for some specific remedies in a six-week course of occupational therapy aimed at my hands. They curl with arthritis, but the middle finger's swollen tendons can't pass through the ligaments, so it triggers up, looking rude to passersby. All the other OT patients come here from keyboards in Silicon Valley, where companies do only half enough to protect the "hands."

Paraffin baths and electric currents in OT fail to untrigger me, so I target my right elbow instead, settling on elective surgery—elective because it's the patient choosing surgery over agony. On operation day I sit in the waiting room beside a soccer player bandaged from knees to Nikes. How nice to be him instead of me with an elbow going lifeless. We're here together because medical practice sometimes marries specialties it ought to separate. Obstetrics with infertility (baby pictures in rooms where women abort and miscarry), and rheumatology with sports medicine. The surgeon in charge, lithe and ruddy, prefers the sports medicine side and admits that laser-scraping the gunk from my joint by arthroscopy "can't do much." He fills out the picture. "Elbow joint completely gone." This is true: my arm quivers reaching for a light switch; I can't point straight at a star. "Disease very, very"—and here comes the ugliest word in doctor language—"advanced."

After the operation the surgeon reports, "Boy, was it depressing in there." For him. No cartilage left, no joint. Bone scraping bone. "And you'll wear out more over time." Soon scar tissue from the surgery shortens the elbow's range, until I can only glimpse my wristwatch by raising an arm to shoulder height. To cheer myself I do this like giving a downbeat, con brio.

Apparently bucking up the spirit can change the body's chemistry. I keep hearing of support groups for breast cancer extending some

women's lives (the brilliant outcome of Dr. David Spiegel's research
at Stanford), so there's no harm trying my clinic's arthritis group. At
my first meeting a doctor explains that old-time strategies began with
low-impact drugs, then worked up the scale. Too bad I'm old-time,
now that they've upended the treatment pyramid. Today's patients take
knockout drugs in the first round to stop arthritis from seizing joints
the way it did mine.

Maybe because of the new treatments every patient here looks peppy,
making me feel like a bag of bones. But before subtracting myself from
the fifteen million Americans in support groups, there's still a stone
to turn. What if I stand *facing* a group? The next day I call Stanford's
arthritis clinic and ask who runs their self-help courses.

"People with arthritis."

"Really. How do *they* get to teach?"

"*You* come to a weekend training session."

In a weekend class of volunteers I train to lead a "self-talk" assignment. I'm to write patients' negative thoughts ("My hands are so
weak," or "My ugly legs limp") on the blackboard—except that I'm
unfit to write on blackboards; they're my farewell to arms. Then the
self-talk point hits home: transform those nasty insults. "No blackboards for me," I chirp aloud. "Scribble your negative thought on these
3 x 5 cards. Then flip them over and rephrase." My card trick proves
a success. We're speaking to ourselves brutally until we flip sides. My
card says:

> **Negative:** I'm so tired. I stupidly nap while everyone else
> gets stuff done.
> **Positive:** Naptime! I've adored it all my life.

After self-talk the class moves on to Why Exercise Works, which
is lost on me, being a body dropout. I tell Kate Lorig, the creator of
Arthritis Self-Help, "Exercise leads to flareups for me."

"Research proves it helps joints, but start small. Walk to the shop-
ping center for lunch." It's fifteen concrete minutes away, and she has
no notion of my legs. On the other hand she's my trainer here. All
afternoon my throbbing feet prove me right, but after that day I actually
alter my bearing. First I start lifting weights, half-pounders: Colgate
tubes. My next goal is to go around a long block on foot, ride my bike a

bit, and swim a couple of lengths: the triathlon. Hard as it is to admit, Arthritis Self-Help is now jiggering my ways, even my joints.

Not long after, in Stanford Medical Center's basement, I teach my own self-help class for fifteen patients, all ages. We start à la AA: "Hi, I'm Mary, and I have RA." Each of us describes what we get from arthritis, its simple gifts:

"Hard time all the time."

"My immune system goes nuts."

"I try everything I can think of, but it just gets worse."

"I have medication and can't stand the stuff."

"Mobility's gone, so what's the future for?"

I hear what I've always thought alone and jot notes in shorthand, nodding like a rabbi. Then one participant pipes up, "How long did you say you had RA?"

"Thirty years."

"Thirty! I'm down one, twenty-nine to go. You don't look bad after all that time."

I have to laugh out loud. In my chronic decline, three decades weaker and running to seed, they see a standout, looking not bad. For them I'm a thing with feathers. I'm hope.

And they give hope too. By the end of six sessions the class has converted the teacher, as I tell my rheumatologist. "Because it's self-help, patients need to want it. Please order your patients to want it."

"Since they feel they're feeling better—"

"It isn't feeling. I saw them revive. One woman just made it to her mailbox until I challenged her to try five more steps. Now she has ten minutes in stride, reaching for eleven." I'm so proud of the movement my class typifies: taking Arthritis Self-Help courses, up to twelve thousand people a year cut pain by a third, doctors' visits almost by half. Not much else alters twelve thousand people in six weeks.

Later I offer a self-help workshop at my clinic, doing my 3 x 5 card trick again. "Anyone want to read a card aloud? The negative and positive sides?" No one volunteers. Then John, in the crowd to support me, raises his hand. Uh-oh. "Negative: Sometimes Mary hurts too much to have sex." Every eye shuttles between us. "Positive: Now I get an erotic kick out of talking with her in bed."

OK. Not bad.

A youngish woman offers to read next. "Negative: I'm tending diabetes every day—shots, strict diet, glucose tests." No positive side comes to mind, but wait, she's flipping her card. "And I'm a control freak, so this is the right disease for me."

Brilliant. It just so happens I too play controller in my household, where I coach everyone's health. Sarah claims I've called white flour a junk food. John points to me as "a moral giant," which may not be the best grade he gives. Alek tells me to chill out, but I say, "Can't let up." Can't let up because I have to micromanage joints. It's the right disease for me, but maybe not for the tribe.

After the workshop the diabetes controller asks me, "What did *you* write on your card?"

"The fear of pain."

"What's on your positive side?"

"That I can see it coming."

What I see coming is already on the way: sequels to RA like thin bones, dry eyes, parched mouth. I'd like to use forewarning as the flip side of fear, but the trouble with bad forecasts, says writer Margaret Gullette about osteoarthritis, is they "make losing seem . . . irresistible." When a bone scan has my physician saying, "Watch out for osteoporosis," I hear a thud. But "you're pretty osteopenic" gives me an adjective to ride on: *bone-poor*. When I tell him, "My eyes feel like beach sand," and he puts a tab of paper under my lids to test for Sjogren's syndrome, losing seems irresistible. He gives me eye drops and a brochure saying that Sjogren's is in cahoots with RA, that it's autoimmune and by the way incurable: it dries out your cells until maybe you can't see, swallow, talk, or perform any of those liquidy functions known as living. But then, a few weeks later, an ophthalmologist takes another eyelid test: "This isn't definitive. Maybe Sjogren's, probably not." Which doc is right? Probably the rheumatologist, but "probably not" is the plot line I'm after. Later a periodontist finds my mouth mingy on bone—RA skips nothing—but still holds me above average ("No lost *teeth*").

The story that I'm vanishing—mouth, bones, liquidity—sets me back to what's-the-point, whereas all I need is to believe myself a decent piece of work.

That's my belief on the last night of '98, when I reach a sore spot inside my back by pressing it over a navel orange. A minute later I feel a touch-and-go of pain and orange juice below my wing, taking these as signs of hard things softening.

Revolution, 1999

In 1999 millennium signs of progress appear everywhere—among them, to my odd delight, one neglected all my years. "Rheumatoid arthritis" is on the shortlist of "new challenges" that the *National Geographic* trusts science will cure. The magazine's reporters ask one patient who applies bee stings to her joints if the treatment bothers her. She has a good answer: "Don't forget I know how arthritis feels." Another day I find "rheumatoid arthritis" in a *New Yorker* piece that names it "the severest of the joint diseases"—not a scoop for a few million sufferers but astonishing news that it's news now. "MANY PEOPLE SUFFER FROM RHEUMATOID ARTHRITIS," declares a late-breaking *New York Times* story, which provides some nasty details:

Their age? More than half under 65.
Working people? More than half of them.
Medication cost? Almost $20 billion in '96 and '97.

These first-ever RA stories in the popular press mark a surprising change: only at the millennium has my disease attracted public consciousness. And the reason? Too many RA patients are dying from gastrointestinal bleeding after taking aspirin or its half-sister ibuprofen, or other nonsteroidal anti-inflammatories. Ironically this side effect from arthritis pills costs more than treating arthritis itself. Too bad I've been popping anti-inflammatories like peanuts, measuring my safety by keeping them near the sink. In fact they give nothing like safety, hospitalizing an estimated twenty-four thousand rheumatoid arthritis patients every year and causing a tenth of those to die. These figures, when I see them, go beyond incredible. Not even tucking aspirin or Advil into buffered coatings or foodstuffs always does the job. The helpful little tablets burn their way right through.

But now a new aspirin replacement claims to block an inflammatory enzyme nicknamed COX-II without attacking the stomach lining. So-called superaspirin is an instant hit, a lamb to lift the pain of the world, or, let's just say, a billion-dollar molecule.

When headlines offer sober medical advice like "MAGIC BULLETS FOR BOOMERS!" or "PLAY ALL DAY," the superaspirin market finds its target demographic, and I'm in it: the seventy-nine million baby boomers moving toward arthritis prime with no mandatory retirement and no dozing at the wheel. Here's a cohort with a screw-that attitude toward pain; here's a breakthrough in pharmacology, an industry looking to profit and an economy strong enough to make "play all day" a reasonable desire.

Arthritis images begin switching so fast I need to hold on. No more old ladies. Now we see Olympian-looking models popping arthritis pills. When a *New York Times* piece shows a peppy woman leaving her laboratory job because her rheumatoid knees can only walk downstairs backward, or when a Harvard doctor laments that half of RA sufferers, mostly women age twenty-five to fifty, in their working-mom prime, have to quit work within ten years of diagnosis, I can hear a click, a recognition that someone's sad private story is socially unfair. A woman doing her job, the women's movement taught us all, shouldn't be stopped by a set of stairs.

"What are you mumbling?" John asks right beside me.

"I'm thinking that feminism raised our expectation of physical fitness and jobs. Whenever an expectation gets noticed by companies, they're sure to sell new drugs."

That night my brother calls from southern California, where he just moved with his wife and teenage daughter. "So, you taking superaspirin yet?"

"My M.D. gave me enough free samples for months, but it's too soon to know if it works."

"What's it called?"

"Celebra at first, then released as Celebrex."

"Why's that?" he asks.

"*Rex* more muscular than *bra*? I'll probably try Vioxx too, a rival drug Merck is dressing for success."

"Good."

"Well, a few tiny concerns. The Food and Drug Administration says the companies haven't *proved* superaspirin safer against stomach bleeding."

"Screw the FDA," says my free-enterprise brother.

"Uh, call you soon."

By popping freebies, patients like me certainly help Celebrex and Vioxx, newborns in '99, corner the huge anti-inflammatory market. Because the companies offer doctors 25 million samples, more than any other class of pill, physicians write "Celebrex" on 2.5 million prescription slips, making it the first drug in history to hit sales of one billion dollars in its infant year. Since the 1997 FDA Modernization Act our watchdog agency also allows drug companies to bankroll clinical trials and push their drugs on my TV. They catch non-arthritis consumers and triple retail sales.

My doctor puts me on another new drug, Arava, launched in '99, the freshest specific RA treatment in a decade. While it inhibits pain-causing inflammatory pyrimidine and stops white blood cells from over-reproducing, it can cause hair loss, diarrhea, liver damage.

Less hair but less pain? Sounds plenty good to me.

Another biotechnology drug for RA comes out in color ads featuring an energetic model and a brash message: "This Is Not the Face of Arthritis." Enbrel "works with your immune system to help control rheumatoid arthritis" by blocking TNF, a tumor necrosis factor that sets off wild alarms. My rheumatologist tells me he walked through a convention where journalists reported Enbrel's "tennis-court-size exhibit" showing "giant x-ray pictures of arthritic joints." As the target for this pitch I'm flattered. Even a drug-resistant strain of patient admires a boundless market. "This is the most exciting time I've witnessed," says a chief FDA adviser. What's exciting to me too: the great drug breakthroughs in '49 and '99 both started with relieving RA, then exploded throughout medicine.

But hypes go along with hopes, as I learned from looking into cortisone. In a headlong rush to drugs it's hard to count hidden costs. Buyers start feeling like beggars, seeing new drugs on TV before they can afford them or receive care. The Arthritis Foundation's medical director advises "early, aggressive treatment" but admits "it's difficult to get early anything when there's not a doctor around." Forty million people with arthritis and related ailments have only thirty-two hundred practicing rheumatologists, roughly half the number needed (Alaska has three), and by 2010 we'll be down to twenty-five hundred, with sixteen million *more* patients. Because our rheumatologists do long-term care, not quick procedures, theirs is the lowest-paid field in internal medicine.

These days I sometimes see Dr. B. in extended appointments shared by fifteen patients instead of waiting for an individual slot. We sit in a circle, pledge not to divulge each other's symptoms, get advice from him or one another, and feel awed by the range of rheumatology—bone diseases, connective diseases, inflammatory and autoimmune diseases, and more. Some of us can't believe we spend *hours* in our doctor's company, and some can't believe we spend hours with others' problems just to have vital signs recorded and a prescription written.

After the group appointment I take my prescription to the clinic pharmacy for my month's supply of Arava and a $250 bill, insurance paid. I know Arava costs five times more than Methotrexate, but for me it works five times better. "How much would Enbrel cost?" I ask.

"Over thirteen thousand dollars annually, but you could save on hospitals down the road."

Turning to the line behind me, I see the 1990s in a nutshell. The average cost of arthritis medicines is thirty-four hundred dollars a year now, and these new-generation drugs go much higher. We're creating two classes of joint owners: those like me, with stable insurance that pays for costly drugs, and those without it, the full-time workers with no benefits, not to mention the part-time workforce, not even to think of the unemployed. They're in line buying Tylenol for their pain.

It seems elementally wrong that bodies should pay twice—once with a malady, once with maldistribution. When the potent pharmaceutical and insurance industries hold back any chance for tax-based care, arguing for the ingenuity of free enterprise, I cheer for ingenuity, even for jumbo profits, but not for a system that keeps other people's joints from my drugs.

At home I scribble "The System" on a notepad, then draw a spider web of companies. American Home Products (Advil) is the major stockholder of Immunex (Enbrel), which is merging with Monsanto and Searle (superaspirin), which coproduces Celebrex with Pfizer. The combined firms promise "a powerhouse in arthritis treatment," reports Wall Street, with billions in market value. I should think so. But who represents the consumer here? Halfway down the page I write "Arthritis Foundation," a great advocacy group that could monitor corporate practices. But here's OrthoLogic sponsoring foundation projects "of interest to OrthoLogic" and other sponsors doing "lifestyle marketing" on the foundation Web site.

As with cortisone in 1949 the system is still sustained by images of victory, expressed in the idea of winning the "pain wars." Cartels run "bruising marketing battles" to produce "smart bombs" that "target the specific components of the immune system" before they "rally more troops" against "the besieged synovial cells" and before TNF can "issue its call for reinforcements." The drugs are "targeting every element of this disease," until joints sound like gunnery zones. This nation's power system is stretching from a military-industrial complex into a promotional-pharmaceutical grid.

On that grid "the profits are outsize, the products unaffordable," I tell my brother on the phone. "But the new drug Arava works wonders, so let's hand cartels credit for rushing great medicines to market." Then I turn to John in the kitchen as I scrub scrambled egg off a pan. "Look what I'm able to do today—wash dishes, take a hike, push a grocery cart, for the first time in years."

"Oh, Mary, it's terrific. It's the drug, right?"

"It's the drug revolution." I lift a pan to a shelf, testing my shoulder. It's still sore. So is the elbow, the ankle. But I'm grateful for separate hotspots instead of all-over fever, for something like a life now. Rising with rising expectations, this Face of Arthritis takes on a skeptical smile and some outside hope.

Ever since I looked for more help from drugs, from surgery, from family, I've also been persuaded by the benefits of hindsight. Now there's a high-level 1999 study in the *Journal of the American Medical Association*, reported in the popular press, that suggests I'm on the right track. Getting help from remembrance makes medical sense. RA patients in the study were asked to write down "the most stressful experience they had ever undergone." Four months later they felt better physically than members of the control group. Dr. David Spiegel (the nation's expert in lengthening survival when cancer patients tell of their anger and grief) interprets these findings about RA: when illness triggers memories of past trauma, "ventilation of negative emotion, even just to an unknown reader, seems to have helped."

That an unknown reader can bring relief merits national news, partly because known listeners make themselves scarce. Apparently chronic patients go knocking, but who's there isn't who they think. "Doctors discourage our stories," writes Anatole Broyard, wanting to chat with his physician about the prostate. I'd like to put a spin on joints, and my doctor listens, but others take seven minutes per appointment, on average, and interrupt a patient's tale after eighteen seconds. Strapped for time, they forward a cultural message: no sickness stories, please.

No sickness stories about arthritis, because this major disease is assumed (wrongly in the case of RA) to be a middling, non-life-threatening disease. Most chronic stories have "no movie version" to entice an audience, quips Margaret Gulette in *Declining to Decline*. No "affirmative ending," says Thomas Couser in *Recovering Bodies*. No plot lines "rendering illness transitory," remarks Arthur Frank in *The Wounded Storyteller*. No twists to keep listeners alert, explains Allison Lurie's novel *The Last Resort*: "That was exactly what Molly's arthritis was like: as if some big old cow had got into her house and wouldn't go away. When other people first became aware . . . they usually began to pretend that the cow wasn't there, and they preferred for Molly to go along with the pretense."

I have reason to believe it's not great to go along with the pretense, a reason my work on genocide lends weight to. Survivors, says psychiatrist Dori Laub, must locate or invent a witness to "enable the unfolding" of life accounts. During the Holocaust Paul Celan revived his murdered mother to address her in a poem, just as Anne Frank made up a friend to hear her diary, and Charlotte Salomon spoke to an imagined "You." On their example I've invented an Angel of Anatomy. I've also written down a "stressful experience" or two, like RA patients in the '99 study, and sometimes I create my own questionnaire:

> What would you say to someone just diagnosed with your
>   condition?
> *Be an agnostic.*

Do you ever have easy times, and what do you make of
    these?
Angel in good mood.

If you pile your worst days all together, what would you not
    throw away?
My widest shoes.

And then I remember Arthur Kleinman's tough question: "Why did
it have its onset precisely when it did?" Personally I leave this one alone.
I won't get near it. The answers I've heard are awful.

John's Aunt Ruth, our feisty relative with RA, says her onset started
with family tragedy. At a party she also tells me, "This is another terrible
year," and I know the terrible she's talking of. But she brightens when
she mentions writing "in a medical journal." I take her to mean a private
diary, but in fact she's sent a short dispatch to her rheumatologist,
which he forwarded to the *Annals of Internal Medicine,* which had the wit
to publish it. Now doctors read of our disease through a patient's eyes,
and a patient gets the benefit of listeners. Now this illness, so severe, so
soundless, is radiantly described: "Pain is the leitmotif of my life. . . .
As for my feet—oh Lord, my feet! I literally haven't taken a single step in
years without pain. . . . I have a distinct physical awareness, even when
my body is still, that it is constantly remembering (echoing may be
the word) the pain of the previous moment and anticipating (sensing,
shadowing) the pain to come. . . . Is my body grossly incapacitated?
Yes, definitely, but just look what it can still do, oh *look!*"

Don't I owe my body that kind of look? To be my own audience for
what it can still do? To watch it, sometimes stumbling and cursing,
through all the curves of a day?

At 9:00 a.m. it can transport me from home to a classroom and prop
me there to teach biography. "A life is lived for itself," I say to the class,
"but a life *history* carries the times." I read from Patricia Williams: "I,
like so many blacks, have been trying to pin myself down in history. I
have been picking through the ruins for my roots." As the class talks
this over, I realize why I've been pinning myself down in history. So
I won't teeter on a narrow outcrop of private experience, I've placed

myself in a larger sequence, seeing a moan-and-groan malady called *rheumatism* turn into a lab-tested disease labeled *arthritis*, then become a social nexus there isn't a name for yet.

That nexus, that new consciousness of illness, will touch each of us in this classroom, each Mexican, Anglo, Polish, Egyptian, Israeli, Chinese person here. Illness unifies sufferers, but now it also bares distinctions. The same lab results in San Salvador or Santa Monica won't play out as the same disease. Now ethnicity and gender, education and income, all distinguish bodies whenever they need repairing. I embody this new meaning of illness, as a midlife, mid-income, mid-campus female, just by walking through a day.

At noon this body navigates campus footpaths toward teaching, thanks to reasonable accommodation (speech-recognition technology, a microphone in my classes, an assistant to carry equipment), available to me because activists objected to segregating the disabled. This body also manages the job because my employer allows me a reduced course load (with a reduced salary that only a two-income household can afford).

Even so, in my next class, drawing a genocide timeline on the blackboard, from "Native Americans" to "African slaves" through "Armenians" up to "Hitler's Reich," my writing arm resists. "I can't write the rest." Subtly the pain that just stopped me shapes what I hear myself saying next: "Ordinary people could have halted Hitler at the start," and I go on from there. "The day that children wouldn't sit near a Jewish child in school, the day a neighbor bypassed the Jewish grocery—small divisions permit huge destructions."

After class I'm thinking that the example is extreme but history works this way, including the history of disability. Where there's segregation, it's perilous to acquiesce.

At 2:35 I walk to the student union, relax my hands around a decaf, and smile on the stunning Malcolm X mural that replaced the anti-Jewish mural painted here before. Stretching my spine, I let some thoughts unwind. Enter the history teacher—with another timeline. I start scribbling (for imaginary students) the progress of America's major ailment, as seen by the witness at hand:

1970s: Pyramid of treatment from weak to strong medicine
  Shifting of social resources to health care
    Search for alternative treatments
      Explosion of women's health movement
        1980s: Terror of immune diseases
          Introduction of early knockout treatments
            1990s: Production of high-performance drugs
              Conversions to self-help
                Demand for disability access
                  Ascent of illness narratives

This long momentum toward more care and public presence has given millions with my disease, and millions with other ones, a safer standing place. Having lived inside these changes, now I see the filaments that tie them to my little stinging joints.

At 3:30 I go up the stairs (elevator broken), tackle the heavy history department door, say "hi" to the chair from a kinder planet (who schedules naptimes between my classes), head to the office, and lie down on my mother's yoga pad. My tired legs feel as if they've trudged through a massive human shift: thanks to vaccines, antibiotics, and public health, people in the developed world now survive fatal infections long enough to acquire lifetime maladies. With my bones flattened on the floor, I realize the new medical revolution has to face diseases that stick. Even AIDS is joining the shift toward lingering ailments. Because the bane of existence has changed from contagious illnesses to chronic ones, a new human condition is here, and arthritis the emblem of it.
One last message flickers before I drop off. The bright American dream is to live widely, then sicken neatly just before passing on. The truth is, we sicken slower, we die longer. Eventually, for millions of us, arthritis is the designated long, slow sickness. We'd be crazy, and we *are* crazy, to think it's someone else's.

4:45. On waking up, something like stubbornness takes hold of me. I look into Alice Wexler's *Mapping Fate* because her brave work on Huntington's chorea both exposes her family disease and opposes acquiescence to it. It helps me see that today (and for years) I've been witnessing arthritis in order to resist it, and not just in myself. My ailment stretches out behind me and will roll on ahead. But first it has to pass *through* me. And I'm not going to let it off easy.

Rights, 1999

If I was saddled with my old despair before new drugs and speech recognition and self-help and resistance, I would not be in Washington in May '99 marching for disability rights or attending a Smithsonian conference where I'd help make feminism user-friendly for disabled people. On one weekend in Washington I reach a juncture of private and public struggles that (I didn't realize) all my moves have been taking me toward. Beyond any shifts in treatment, attitudes, or technology, beyond any steps that have gotten me this far, I discover a new way to identify myself with my malady. In fact I reverse the way I've done it before.

After crossing the country, I start by phoning Simi Linton, whose book *Claiming Disability* urges disabled people to own their distinctiveness. "How do I find you at the march?"

"Any visual impairment?" she says straight off. "No? Then I'm white. I'm in a red mobilized power chair. I'm wearing brown pants."

So this is disability identity: forthright about color, no-nonsense about aids, uncowed about handicaps. In one instant I switch my own marker from "able-bodied" to "nondisabled," which gives disability the front row I've been shooing it from. An hour later I find Simi near a song leader who's calling, "I'll sing, then you sing or sign back to me." Around us people are rollicking through a song in American Sign Language while moving toward the Supreme Court to tell the justices, Don't you dare weaken the Americans with Disabilities Act. At the head of the line a man lifts prosthetic arms in a presidential V, as in, "Here we come, Air Force One."

Suddenly a woman lawyer, swinging her briefcase and blunt-cut hair, strides right across our line. "Feminism got you here," my anger says. "Pay some respect to the next cause." For the first time I'm proud of my own halting gait, the right speed for the wheelchairs around me.

"No barriers, no boundaries, no bullshit," we chant at the Supreme Court steps, some through bullhorns, some through ventilators. And: "Most integrated setting means most integrated setting." I should know what I'm chanting about, so I ask a wheelchaired Vietnam vet to explain. He says the ADA orders states to provide disabled services in "the most integrated setting" and hands me a leaflet from the militant group ADAPT (Americans Disabled for Attendant Programs Today). I learn of a right I haven't seen before as a right: to receive services at home with relatives around you. I read about the Supreme Court's '99 *Olmstead* decision, condemning "unjustified isolation . . . as discrimination based on disability." I now know that nineteen states call the ADA and *Olmstead* unconstitutional, including California.

"So if the Court favors those states, can my employer stop complying with the ADA?"

"That's what the chants are about," the vet says. They're about the right to reasonable accommodation at any job, the right to decent elevators and clerical aids at mine.

Simi and I head off after the rally, but a block from the high court we come on a woman waiting in full sun for a wheelchair van that hasn't come. Up until now I would have said, That kind of problem isn't mine. Impairments like hers appear inherent, whereas mine feels unstable, with symptoms flaring up, vitality coming and going. My disease seems less definitive, less marked than a disability. And I don't want to be marked.

I also figure the feeling is mutual. Right here on the streets feisty people in wheelchairs prove disability is *not* a disease, does not invite quarantine or require cure. It seems to me the ill and disabled fear each other's stigmas, stay at arms' length, arguing over the beginnings and the ends of life. From long experience of illness and pain I find I'm for aborting a fetus with severe and fatal genetic problems and also for controlling the choice to die. But people with disabilities have good reason to fear selective amniocentesis with abortion (in case it's used against tolerable disablements) and dismiss the choice-to-die (in case someone else makes the choice to get rid of them).

Setting myself on a curb for a moment, I feel bound to the illness side. Then I notice my stiff and achy legs. Actual bodies get disabled from being sick and sick from being disabled. Wouldn't it make sense, after all, to embrace a conflicted double identity?

At the next day's conference, however, I'm taken for what I seem at first glance, a nondisabled feminist historian (no wheelchair, no signing). Fine with me. My presentation gladly asserts that disability rights draw on feminist insights, that sex and impairment come from biology while gender and disability take cues from society. "We all embody gradations of genes and of experience that society segregates into two distinct genders or abilities. Only prejudice makes impaired people *disabled*," I hear myself remark, as if these "people" were someone else. As a nondisabled feminist I'm pleased to derive this other movement's chant, "Nothing about us without us," from feminism. Like my own movement, disability rights must broaden to countries where four hundred million disabled people live outside the distribution of medicine and services, a deep underclass—maybe the most deprived people on an abundant earth.

An hour later at a restaurant my distance from "this other" movement bites the dust. We have four wheelchairs at the table, two people signing, and someone with RA who can't talk over the sound system. Finally I ask the waitress, "Could you possibly turn the music off?" She looks uncertain. "A few of us," I say, "are hard of hearing."

"You hard of hearing?" someone at the table signs.

"No, I'm hard of speaking"—I make up that term right then. "My vocal cords," I confess a little proudly, "are stiffened, like my arms." Aha, I've announced myself: I'm *not* nondisabled. Granted, it takes awhile (a minute) for anyone to notice my off-angle hands, my style of speaking low. Granted, I get by without showing a body-based identity, and I'm not yet a woman waiting for a wheelchair van. But from this moment I want to number myself among Americans with Disabilities.

What's bringing about the change? It's because I feel at ease here, seeing and joining, yes, a renewed civil rights struggle, captured by a handmade wheelchair sign: I CAN'T EVEN GET TO THE BACK OF THE BUS. Arthritis sufferers speak of joints, not rights. We're part of a medical problem, not a political movement. If we're lame, we don't claim lame. We don't "stare back," as disabled people describe the new look. We don't acknowledge we're stared *at*. We don't brood over the "unfit," denied visas or work. From a towering disease we don't scan vistas of history to locate our place in it.

But we ought to. All of us with arthritis, alone and invisible, could form a social cause. And if we called out our needs—public health for chronics, coverage for long-term care, rheumatologists everywhere, research on connective-tissue diseases, support for the NIH and the Arthritis Foundation—then we arthritis people could offer the disability community millions of bodies to count politically with theirs. Plus we could contribute one four-letter word: pain. Disability rights announces empowerment. But the challenge of human suffering? Not in the chanting yet.

An hour later, as this formerly nondisabled feminist walks slowly back from the restaurant to the alabaster gleam of our high court, I don't want a benevolent society—just a just one. I can't apologize anymore for the trouble I cause, my need of assistance, equipment, quiet in public places. Before the new century I'd shout (if my voice could) from the Supreme Court's bottom step: Make a way for me. It's the law.

Home in the kitchen I start telling John, "I'm not alone anymore. I'm surrounded by the disabled. They've handed me a new identity." He touches my shoulder, and I go on. "Before, I felt like a fall-behind—not always my fault, but still below the mark. To be ill *and* disabled is to be myself and also make a fuss."

John's quick smile encourages me. So I spread the word to my brother: "I just marched in Washington," and to please him I add, "Like you in the sixties."

"We're not so different, Mary."

Then I call my friend Ruth. "In DC I got a different picture of myself. For the first time being slow-gaited and soft-voiced made me *belong*."

"That's a pretty significant change."

"It feels that way. People with disabilities show so much courage searching for rights and recognition, they make me want to become a shaker and mover."

"So you want to be noticed even if your illness isn't?"

"I do. Announcing I've got so-called unsightly arthritis—and that's who I am—reminds me of coming into feminism in the seventies, making private issues political, redefining what's normal if a woman like me feels abnormal."

Ruth pauses a minute, then says, "You just renamed a disorder into a disability."

"Right. And you know what? Disability isn't a state. It's a continuum I'm on. So are a lot of others, and we're letting go of shame."

Owning disability turns out to be a summit marker, added to others: Sarah's thirtieth birthday and two graduations—hers with an M.A. and Alek's from high school. On a flight to celebrate in Seattle, John seats me beside his long legs in an emergency row, but really, lifting an exit door is asking a lot of someone who can't break into her airline pretzels. From another row I watch him open his backpack, pull out a German or Spanish poem to translate, then organic carrots and raw broccoli— his typical meal that others have called Gandhiesque. Alek squashes into the next seat with his total baggage—two clarinets, nineteen hip-hop CDs, and one change of T-shirt should the need arise. At SeaTac airport Sarah greets us with the patient enthusiasm she uses teaching preschool—"changing the world," she says, "ten kids at a time"— while Scobie pulls everyone into a hug and shoulders all the baggage. They open their car trunk, pushing aside Yale band newsletters Sarah wants to give Alek, brochures for her early-childhood workshops, kites that Scobie has designed.

Then there's me to deal with, the one who can't carry a carry-on, who clings to Alek's arm. "You OK, Ma?" he asks. "Yep," I say and lose my grip on a purse, a ticket, a friend's book on the Congo. At that same instant I release a piece of my life, a piece keeping RA under wraps. I've seen my son through senior year, my daughter to her profession and her partner. I've seen my parents to paradise, my brother to Pasadena, my drugs transformed, my rights announced, my identity reset. I've seen thirty years without RA, thirty years with it. High time to graduate.

Then everyone points up to Mount Rainier, cut by clouds, needing nothing but new visions to top it.

Hands, 1999

After the dazzle of Rainier certain flashes of awareness seem to enter the atmosphere. This is the only way to describe what I'd call a conversion.

I've been moving like a pilgrim through stations I see clearly now—getting hurt by arthritis, then getting wise to it, then getting help for it. If there's further movement in store, and I think there is, it will probably come (as it has before) with journeys and with losses, until at the end I have more wisdom in my hands.

"Paris," John says as the airport shuttle takes us past Notre Dame.

Nod.

"What's the matter? I thought you wanted to be here. *Paris.*"

"I did." I don't now, though we signed up to teach a Stanford course on wartime France. "It's the cathedrals." Stone floored. "The bistros." Loud. The air of excitement. Cold.

But gradually I warm to the baker and stationer and the clothing shops on our street, to the outdoor *marché biologique* where we trek every week for organic food. One day we find an ornate library in our neighborhood where I rest my feet most afternoons and look up female authors. That's when I'm forced to discover a new side to them. Madame de Sévigné, famous letter writer, confesses in 1676 that rheumatism cuts her off: "I cannot close my hand. . . . I cannot use [it] to write." Novelist George Sand mentions "cruel attacks of rheumatism" disabling her right arm. Her friend Flaubert warns that her "bathing in streams very likely is the cause," missing a more probable cause—that the disease routinely seizes the device writers write with. What else can we do but use our hands and endanger what they're good for?

This awful question makes me wish for fewer parts to lose. I search out a famous Apollo in the Louvre, without any limbs for centuries.

When Rainer Maria Rilke saw one like it, its torso dazzled him into writing his famous line: "You must change your life."

I'll give that a try.

I take off with John and Alek to sun-ripened Provence, with a guide-book to "inns of charm and distinction." One night we reach an un-marked inn while a torrent paints the place black. We're put in a cellar with bunks that the innkeeper guards by locking us in. When Alek, shivering and soaked, dares turn on an ancient lamp, he crashes to the floor, shocked but not quite fried. The next day, after a shower whose charm and distinction soak the whole room, we respectfully ask why the inn has no outside light, no sign, no shower curtain, no shock-free lamp, no adult bed, no unbarred exit. Instead of saying with sorrow, "It's a dungeon, you see," the innkeeper draws up and proudly announces, "C'est le plan."

In three words she changes my views. Whatever seems imprisoning belongs to an absurd design. So let arthritis cause screwups, loosening my grip on a plate or throttling my voice in a lecture. From now on I'll concede to the Angel of Anatomy, "That's the plan." That's what I'm given to work with in this life.

Then I hear of a famous surrealist artist who lived in France for decades and painted exactly the Angel I've been trying to envision. With her penetrating eyes and world-encompassing wings she stops at nothing, either to help or to hurt. Her exposed joints fit into their skeletal sockets with a strength she won't conceal. L'Ange d'Anatomie, by Leonor Fini, materializing in 1949 (the cortisone moment of hope), fiercely takes the viewer past the edge of certainty into uncontrollable fate. An Angel of Anatomy is nothing less than the power an imagina-tion creates to name the world's reckless dispatch of health or death.

With that potent figure in mind I settle back into Paris, put myself on-line, hit "Open New Mail," and find this:

> health diagnosis is the pits. terminal cancer of the liver.
> prognosis something in range of 6 months to 1.5 yrs. w/o
> possibility of cure

No capitals, no lead-up or cool-down, no signature, which means it's from my brother.

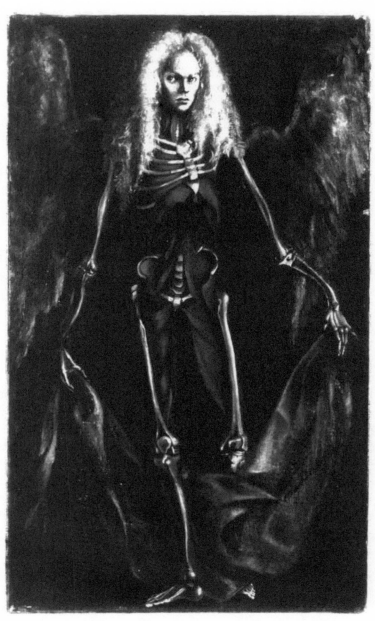

Leonor Fini, L'Ange d'Anatomie, 1949. Courtesy of the Leonor Fini Estate.

"Listen," I say by long distance. "Don't stop being . . ."

"What?"

Don't stop being my brother, I want to say, but I retreat to what people ask about terminal illness: "Who's your doctor?"

A few days later by e-mail:

scan also reveals cirrhosis

My chain-smoking brother who only drank Coke has clear lungs and cirrhosis? Is the Angel nuts?

my spirits are fine, except for growing depression about the deterioration of my bridge game

"You're still the best player. The thing to guard against is any hint you earned this illness. It just happens."

yeah, going the way our dad went (just like that, while having a haircut) is a better deal but i admit it IS a luxury to be able to prepare for one's own demise

"Prepare, yes, like the singer Charles Trenet here: 'Those coming to my last concert are excused from coming to my funeral.' And soon I'll send you some tips I picked up from Renoir."

Museum to museum I'm searching for artwork by Pierre Auguste Renoir, painted in the grip of rheumatoid arthritis. Struck at age fifty, debilitated at sixty, almost completely disabled at seventy, with all his bones poking through the skin, so disfigured he couldn't wear shoes, with hands swollen like my hands, without strength to turn a door-knob, his fingers "stuck together," a friend said, "against the palm of his miserable hands, fleshless, like the legs of poor chickens"—Renoir set his mind to do just one thing. Wedging a brush in his fingers, hand-kerchiefs around his wrist, reaching his canvas by cranking it up and down, inventing a mobile easel from a bicycle chain, he just made art.

One day in front of a Renoir painting my breath slows at how in-sidiously rheumatoid arthritis shows through. I see he shortened his brushstrokes and thinned the oils against the effort.

Yet I also catch the astonishing way his works grew more sensuous. Instead of darkening each *nature morte*, he painted still-lifes with the

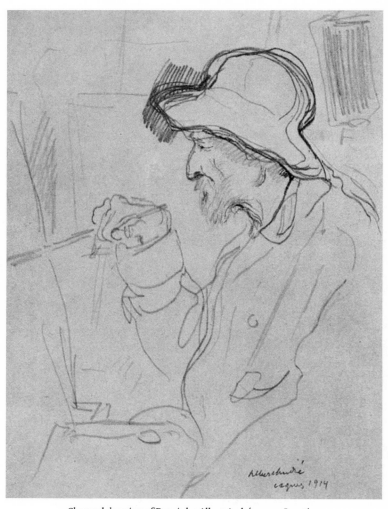

Charcoal drawing of Renoir by Albert André, 1914. Location
unknown. Courtesy of the municipality of Cagnes-sur-Mer.

freshness of stems leafing out, a radiance pushing through the skins of
onions like heat through his own skin. His dealer Vollard saw him set
off "groaning to the studio," but Renoir said, "You see, Vollard? One
doesn't need hands to paint. They're quite superfluous." To a collector
he announced, "Really, I am a lucky man. Now I can do nothing but

paint." Extremely ill, he depicted a garden of delights, always believing, "We must embellish!" At the last hour in 1919, still outflanking pain, he called for brushes, paints, and flowers. And then: "I think I begin to make something out of it all."

Tracing Renoir's condition, I panic about my brother's. "Should I fly home and force him to take treatment, even though it probably won't help?"

"What does he say he wants?" Alek asks quietly.

"To keep going without chemo as long as he can play bridge."

"Is he clear about it?"

"Absolutely clear."

"Then that's your answer."

Alek watches over me, John watches over me, my friend Marilyn, stopping in Paris, watches over me and lets me say, "All these years my brother bullied me and misused his body, but I was the one to get sick. And now—"

"Now is for forgiveness."

"How odd that he's the one to bring from extreme illness—clarity. It's the thing I never thought of. He keeps his skill firmly in hand and waives the desire to outlive it." Then I rush away in need and dread of another e-mail. It turns out to be the final one:

> i will write one last short piece, to be published posthu-
> mously, entitled "Bridge as Praise for God"

He's come to the moment Renoir reached, exactly eight decades earlier, saying, "I think I begin to make something out of it all." My brother dies suddenly in December, as my mother, my father, and Renoir did. By way of obituary he gets his dream, an entire Bridge Column in the *New York Times*, calling him "one of the most imaginative and creative personalities in the world of bridge."

On a plane from Paris to Pasadena for his memorial service I switch from knowing to remembering him: how he stunned Sarah by playing Beethoven so loud his new stereo exploded, how he tickled Alek by discussing Mahler at four in the morning. From now on these memories come back without him.

The next time I visit his wife and daughter they ask if I'd like to see where his ashes rest. Their church is soft lit, with gilded crosses

marking vaults like safe deposit boxes, and I know my no-faith, free-
enterprise brother must be getting a kick out of that.

Outside with his best friend and bridge partner, all I can say is, "Have
you played since my brother . . . ?"

"One tournament without him."

"That's wonderful." Without him.

"It wasn't bridge."

"Why not?"

"Because, Mary, your brother was the best bridge partner in the
world."

I'm at a loss for words. Best partner is the best a person can be.
Finally I say, "His spirit is in there. It really is."

"He was speaking to you?"

"To all of us. He says, *Play your hand.*"

And that settles my vision. Suddenly I feel better for all that has come to
me—dazzling drugs, publicity for RA, a forceful disability movement,
a faith in my family as odd and OK, a journey. I'm grateful for getting
help from medicine, from feminism, from family and friends, from
politics and pharmaceuticals. But it's a curled hand ("One doesn't need
hands") that tells me how to live for writing, like my brother's hand
for cards or Renoir's with a brush. In losses they kept their skills, their
passions, and for these gave praise.

Later I find an unopened e-mail on my brother's computer, the
last message I'd sent him. It's about Renoir on his deathbed, about
getting past the body's final constraints. His ultimate request: "Don't
let them lay too heavy a stone" over agonized arthritic limbs, "so I'll
have strength to lift it if caught by desire to roam the land."

V. Getting Past

we will wear new bones again
Lucille Clifton, *"new bones"*

Healing

My brother remembered, at the last, to play whatever hand was dealt, showing me how the game goes, how to place each turn on top of earlier ones and honor where they came from.

The hands dealt by arthritis, I've learned, aren't half so hard as they once were. The fact that many RA patients are ending up less disabled than I am, now that they take power-packed medicines at the disease's outset, counts as a fine deal. But arthritis still brings losing hands too. It still dislodges thousands of people from lives they'd like to live or outflanks all the medication tried on it. Too many are missing insurance or access to drugs and doctors. While pain damages their bodies, women more than men get used to bearing it, or if they demand that doctors take it away, as Melanie Thernstrom reports, this is "misinterpreted as hysteria." And 2005 research confirms what no one's supposed to tell, that people with RA are more likely to die a decade earlier than others, that women with RA have shorter lifespans than men with RA and have two times more heart attacks than other women.

Still, I've been praising my deal since 2003, when the great biologic drug Enbrel started helping me jog and hike and cook and write a sentence by hand for the first time in years. But drug makers gain returns four times above average (as my friend Ruth writes in her newspaper column), while their products stay proprietary and unaffordable. Enbrel carries a monthly tab of thirteen hundred dollars and a long list of side effects, "including death." Like cortisone, miracle drugs knock down more than they're meant to, as in Steve Martin's lampoon of a fantasy pill for joint pain: "Side effects: This drug may cause joint pain."

Side effects from the superaspirin Vioxx, which I (along with 25 million others) swallowed for years, were suspected from the outset,

namely increased risk of heart attack and stroke. But neither the FDA
nor the manufacturer conducted specific clinical trials or added a "black
box warning." After five lucrative years Merck pulled the drug in 2004,
while medical watchdogs berated its executives for hiding the risks
and roasted the government for depending on company research. This
case sets a dangerous precedent for drug makers to stretch the market,
"pitch the products far beyond the ranks of arthritis patients to people
with more ordinary aches," conceal adverse side effects, provide foun-
tains of free samples, take profits early—and then fend off regulations
and lawsuits by withdrawing their drug. Suddenly patients with serious
arthritis (who might choose well-known risks in exchange for benefits)
lose the medication entirely. When I think of these patients going back
to aspirin, a remembrance of taking twenty ineffectual aspirin a day
makes me laugh until I cough.

It's heartening when over-the-counter alternatives like glucosamine
and chondroitin repair cartilage, as the best-selling *Arthritis Cure* claims.
But call it a loss that these pricey "supplements" (like other unregulated
pills) empty millions of wallets, or that Coca-Cola tests them in a bev-
erage boasting "Joy for Joints." It's good to know that taking common
vitamins like C and D lowers the risk of getting RA (cigarettes heighten
it), but large doses of vitamin C can provoke serious osteoarthritis.
It's helpful to read research showing how weight-loss-plus-exercise
reduces pain from osteoarthritis, but it's still perverse that remarkably
few studies have assessed the low-priced effects of good nutrition. It's
good that long-term breast-feeding wards off RA, but the reverse seems
to hold for those who already have the disease.

Neither the good news nor the bad has lifted arthritis beyond its
history of humility. For reasons I've uncovered along the way—its
commonness, its incurability, its association with lower-status groups
(women, elders), its stigma of recession—a serious, dominant, sometimes deadly disease still stays muted in our culture. Now the shame
is that medical schools barely push the skills of lifelong care, though
chronic diseases sicken almost half our population and suck up four-
fifths of healthcare expenses, with osteoarthritis alone distressing at
least sixteen million American women and five million men. It also
doesn't help that today's doctors depend on computerized codes more

than patients' life histories. Still, some are starting to practice "narrative medicine," analyzing illness stories for clues.

Count it as a step forward that someone like me can now dictate stories about RA. But while other writers boot up their word processors, my speech-recognition program crashes on terms like *narrative medicine*. Not long ago I got so impatient I called the manufacturer.

"Hi. I need to replace some software?"

"I'm sorry. We're not shipping at present."

"How 'bout tomorrow?"

"I'm afraid we're in Chapter Eleven."

"But I didn't get to chapter 11!"

It's a bad sign when fraud arrives via the phone or when I backtrack through Wall Street reports on Dragon Systems' speech-recognition monopoly, finding falsified sales, cooked-up earnings, unaudited loans, a CEO pocketing twenty-five million dollars, and finally a bankruptcy that interrupted crucial technology and left this end user struggling.

It's shocking too when the CDC begs the nation "to focus on arthritis as a public health problem," numbering Americans with the disease at seventy million—"too big to ignore"—but the government operates the National Institute of Arthritis and Musculoskeletal and Skin Diseases on five hundred million dollars, less than 2 percent of the total NIH budget.

Call it hopeful that citizens keep taking public action, as when Arthritis Foundation members mailed thirty thousand empty pill bottles to Congress with the message: cover medicines with Medicare. Also hopeful that California has finally dropped its lawsuit against the Americans with Disabilities Act. But call it dreadful that our nation's highest court prevents state workers like me from suing for compliance with the ADA, ruling that "discrimination against employees with disabilities . . . does not violate the Constitution"—a judgment to howl at, an ominous precedent allowing states to cancel *any* equal protection of the laws.

Call it a low hand that I'm still being hurt by heavy doors and broken elevators on my state campus. Call it better that a lawsuit is forcing my school to spend five million dollars on upgrades, not to mention an Institute on Disability founded by my colleague Paul Longmore. Call it a high point when a conference on disabled women (assembled by my friend Mary Rothschild in Arizona) lets students with RA speak their feisty minds. I hear one of them say, "My arthritis shows my children how to handle a life with limits"—a side effect I never actually thought of. Another student, with a new baby, is asked, "Does your wheelchair bother your husband?" and answers, "Uh, evidently not." Then a third states, "I used to be a mind attached to a body, but here at college I become a body attached to a mind." That's it. That sums up my rapture with education. It took me years to learn this one thing: what is good for tackling a chronic condition isn't knowledge, it's pursuit of knowledge.

In this pursuit I still see arthritis as a disease of losses, but I'm getting past a few of them. I'm moving beyond my deficit ABCs—Arthritis, Boredom, Concealment—and in fact expanding my alphabet. When Alek walks in from his summer job and asks, "What're you doing?" I say, "Finding words for joints that start with W-X-Y-Z."

A minute later Alek brings me *Leaves of Grass*. "Walt Whitman, two Ws," he says and shows me a passage he loves:

> And your very flesh shall be a great poem and have the
> richest fluency not only in its words but in the silent lines
> of its lips and face and between the lashes of your eyes and
> in every motion and joint of your body.

"Oh, Alek, it's the essence. The richest fluency not only in words but in joints. I'm so grateful."

Later I tell John, "I'm getting back to the last time I had fluency in every motion and joint."

"What a beautiful phrase."

"It's Whitman's. Alek found it for me." It implies that fluency in speaking counteracts loss of fluency in motion, and the shame of loss.

Later that night John has occasion to lose fluency in motion too: he suffers a back spasm, brought on by lugging my sources (old journals and letters and photos) back to the attic. While he lies still as bronze, Alek and I scurry to help, until Alek too tumbles down, with a fever. For two days I play nurse for extra-strength menfolk until they totter to their feet and RA tosses me back to my side of the ward.

Then I feel voided out. The short and long jobs of caring are over
for now. Alek's off to another year of college, maybe never returning
to live nearby. "Remember years ago sending Sarah to college," John
says, "then rushing from the airport to get Alek at daycare?"

I remember. Now every time Alek heads away, the sorrow of missing
Sarah comes back too. I put a hand on John's spine. "And I'm supposed
to store those child-filled years in the attic, with everything I don't need
anymore?" Late that night I wait up, for memory's sake, to catch a last
glimpse of Alek asleep on my couch, his limber frame folded at angles,
his head turning to mumble, "'Night, Ma."

What feels so empty now? I ask myself when he leaves. Not having
him here? Not being a daily mother? I bite into a bagel at a computer-
buzzing coffee shop. Not being able to renew myself, because of my
joints? Two gulps of decaf. Not seeing any way past RA? I rush home to
find an antique volume from a Paris bookstall. It might help.

Voyage around My Room seems to foreshadow my present state of
mind and offer a plan. In 1794 France, Xavier de Maistre suffered strict
house arrest, which he made bearable by circling his room inch by inch,
recording a careful history of its holdings. I've started to do the same:
"This pen was a present from Alek. This pillow I stitched in honor of
Sarah being born . . ." Xavier de Maistre concluded, "All this would
make even the most indolent person inclined to start writing." When
his time was served, the voyage came full circle to the starting place.
Now he could see, and write, his history freshly, from another side.

After hearing Whitman's "fluency . . . in every motion and joint of
your body," I've lighted on this X. Like Xavier de Maistre I've traveled
around a constricted periphery for years—ah, there's my Y: years with
RA. As for Z . . . it should be zero gravity, a state I've finally arrived
at, suspended between physical drag and the upward lift of ideas. The
first time I heard of zero gravity, in '69, I was holding month-old Sarah
in front of a fuzzy TV as astronauts touched the moon. That moment
circles back now, through joint memory.

Another gravity-lifting moment circles back too. Eyeing distant Mount
Rainier several years ago and looking for new vision, I never hoped
to hike that sky-high place. Now I've come here, along with Ruth and
Sarah and Scobie and John, who's pulling me up the steep trails and

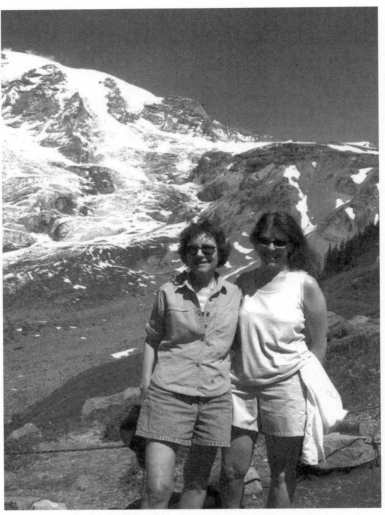

Mary and Sarah at Mount Rainer, Washington, 2004. Photo by Scobie Puchtler.

lifting me back down. On each hike I grow more certain that arthritis touches most of my body but only a fraction of my being, even smaller when I'm with people I love. As I call up moments from the past—say, Sarah playing the flute and Alek the clarinet—I remember attending to my children first, then to my disease. I'm beginning to own this illness by understanding it never owned all of me. Up on the mountain we talk of this as we never have before.

"I just wanted to be a parent and a person, not a patient," I tell my family.

"With the result that we all maintained a culture of silence," says Sarah, "around the fact and the pain of your arthritis."

Yes, they carried the fact and the pain at some deep and quiet level. Even some of my close friends hardly knew. "But that culture of silence wasn't just ours," I say. "Around arthritis it existed everywhere. In my case the disability movement finally cut through it." As we stop for a huddle-like hug, a love-bunch, I see that my getting onto this mountain has taken the combined efforts of family and friends, along with great medication and an astute doctor. But the new vision I have here—that I finally want to be just what I've become—required a long journey around my joints, every step of the way. It's what I call healing by history.

After Rainier I hike the hills behind Stanford as if I'm walking along my timeline. I recall the spot where a kite lifted my spirit, helped me look back on myself. And the place where I stumbled on a tiny stone, fell full-length into third grade and remembered the joints of dinosaurs. These hills are where I began believing that history could do a body good. For the time being (and that's all the time I'll count on) I reach the Endurance Tree with more ease than years before. I'm even ready to push further, all the way to the starting place.

There's one more question to get past, the one I haven't wanted to ask.

Why, at the outset, did rheumatoid arthritis happen to me?

The truth is, I've never seen any reason why not me. I've spent a career studying genocide, and I was spared that. Why should I be spared a joint disease?

I shouldn't be. As I look over the past, "Why me?" goes so far beyond me it looks like a procession stretching through millennia, from Greek physicians to high-tech doctors, from Roman legions to pain researchers, from rheumatism to autoimmunity. Expanding the scope of my disease is how history healing works for me. It proves that even the cause of arthritis keeps changing over time. What used to be favored—humors, airs, infections—gave way to psychosexual disorders, immune cells, carbohydrates in the cartilage. Finally it's clear why one true cause has never been pinned down: simply because there are so many of them. The question "Why me?" can only sort out which cause I *believed* and what I believe now.

Deep in the overstuffed armchair where I've hugged each baby and sat stupefied by pain, I'm holding the source for an answer in two sentences. One comes from an old letter to my sister-in-law Susan, saying of my first pregnancy, "I'm crackling with health." I didn't *have* any problems before those trimesters in 1969. So it's childbirth I have to return to, figuring out what started there.

The other sentence comes from the journal of scientist Dorothy Hodgkin, explaining the onset of her RA at the same age as my onset (twenty-eight) but years before: "I found myself very stiff and aching in every joint. Rheumatoid arthritis, acute." She called herself "a typical case: a young woman, under some stress"—stress from a tough first childbirth and a newborn's ill health. Hodgkin's "typical case" passes into me like an old family story. And that's just it: the story's so familiar. Here and there for years women have told me that rheumatoid arthritis sprang on them with a first child.

At my doctor's a week later I come straight to the point: "Dr. B., have you seen lots of women whose RA started at maternity?"

"I've seen it, yes, but not that much research about it."

"And I've heard women's stories, but not that much fuss."

The next weeks I spend in a medical library, discovering what most researchers dwell on: the fact that already existing RA improves during pregnancy and that often the improvement doesn't last. But they devote much less study to whether childbirth *causes* a rheumatic condition or how one birth could prompt a lifelong disease. Into this knowledge-gap slips Dorothy Hodgkin's suspicion that stress from childbirth itself (physical? mental?) touches off "rheumatoid arthritis, acute."

Eventually Hodgkin's hands became gnarled with RA, but they accepted the Nobel Prize for chemistry in 1964; they received the British Order of Merit in 1965; they deciphered insulin in 1969; and over time they grew, she said, "more and more like the picture," a piercing portrait of arthritic hands drawn by the sculptor Henry Moore. In '69

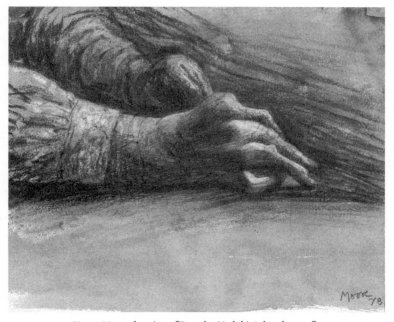

Henry Moore drawing of Dorothy Hodgkin's hands, 1978.
Reproduced by permission of the Henry Moore Foundation.

Hodgkin had more fame than any woman in science, yet science didn't know why her hands had RA.

In '69 I too became, in Hodgkin's words, a "typical case: a young woman, under some stress," ending up with her disease. To grasp this now I have to reopen my old beliefs. One was that RA originates from physical changes during pregnancy. The other was that it derives from coming "under some stress" afterward.

For some years I assumed that my mostly female disease stemmed from female hormones. Now in the medical library I peer closer. Yes, femaleness is the *prime* risk factor for RA. But if hormones produce autoimmune disease, it turns out they do it deviously. During pregnancy, when they gather force for nine months, RA actually relents. And of course RA shows up in women without pregnancy and in men too. So my first assumption was off: female hormones aren't a straight-line cause.

I've also imagined a kind of allergic reaction, as if pregnancy made me itch or sneeze. Medical studies go along with this idea: pregnant bodies can recoil when sperm bring guest DNA—say, for instance, John's genes. Actually I don't want to think this, don't want him to think this, but I can't get past it. Without DNA from him, would I have RA?

With this question I have to walk outside, past the Endurance Tree and every spot in the hills that opened a memory stile, all the way to a high view of San Francisco Bay where I can release the simplistic idea that John did me in. Up here there's a more intricate story to consider.

It seems that a kind of allergic reaction actually flows from the fetus. Its HLA antigens, the ones that tell self from nonself, create antibodies in the pregnant woman. These antibodies cause remission of RA, as they did before Alek's birth, because a pregnant woman's immune cells work so hard against fetal HLA that they abandon their usual job of attacking joints. But such antibodies can also cause a dramatic relapse after pregnancy.

What's becoming clear is that a reaction between self and non-self involves identity. If the pregnant woman and fetus have look-alike molecules (suggests Dr. J. Lee Nelson, a researcher in Seattle, where Sarah now lives), "the maternal immune system apparently gets con-fused: which is real, and which the impostor?" Intrigued, I check my notes to be sure. Right there. The maternal immune system gets nervous about the identity of the fetus.

Now identity, as cutting-age studies say, is multiple. The identity confusing my own immune system might have formed in the sperm or the fetus . . . or somewhere else?

Back to the medical library. There new findings take my breath away. It turns out that genetic material, crossing the placenta both ways, leaves long-term consequences. Packs of cells from the fetus drift around a mother for years after her child's born. And fetal cells cause a sort of graft-versus-host disease, kept active by autoimmune reactions in the mother's body. In other words my first child's cells may still be curdling with my own. But it's not exactly a case of hers versus mine. Mine also include maternal cells that crossed the placenta to me in 1941. "It's a uniquely female risk to have these transgenerational effects," says Dr. Nelson.

So it's possible my newborns weren't "allergic" to me alone but to my mother. And that my body's reaction was not to them but to some triple alliance of their cells and John's cells and maybe his mother's. Good lord.

At last my suspicion—that RA arrived directly, prenatally, allergenically, from everyone closest to me—blanches as I focus current knowledge on it. So many other agents came into play: genes inherited from parents, antibodies and hormones flooding the body during pregnancy, plus environmental factors uncounted yet (remarkably few studies have been done on viruses, pollutants, or diet). And even these prenatal conditions prompting an autoimmune illness are not the final word.

To keep exploring, I borrow decades of American Rheumatology Association reports from Dr. B. and find out what physicians believed at the time of my RA onset. They believed in slow and cautious treatment of a sudden disease. Aspirin alone would combat new RA, along with "rest, modification of activities" rather than exercise. Long before they upended the treatment pyramid, doctors warned each other to postpone cortisone ("a year of steroid therapy is roughly equivalent to four years of normal aging") and to keep mortality in mind: both RA and its treatment, they stressed, carry "major complications leading to death." As I'm reading what was in store for me, I stumble on a revealing coincidence. The very day I went into labor in June '69, my future doctor, on the way to his new job, delivered a research talk on immune reactions in rheumatoid arthritis. As I headed to the clinic he was about to join, he addressed the disease I was about to acquire. This coincidence underlines a question I'm now putting to the test. Did RA actually arrive *after* pregnancy, namely, while I was giving birth?

Since that's when newborn jaundice also appeared, was jaundice part of RA onset? And was the miscarriage ending my second pregnancy also linked to RA—or to hot tubs women weren't warned against? Why was the third pregnancy dogged by newborn jaundice and flareups again? Since RA accompanied this whole reproductive sequence, was I responsible for all of it?

Starting with jaundice, I check Medline databases every which way, but no one suggests causal links between RA and this newborn condition. Studies only confirm that mothers stay fearful for their jaundice-born babies long afterward, which I wish I'd known then. As for miscarriage, research proves that RA does increase the risk. At least it wasn't the hot tub: not my fault. Flareups with childbirth? Here's another finding I didn't know about till now. Pregnancy cools a woman's immune system so she doesn't throw out the baby with the bathwater, but afterward the coolers, or immune suppressors, slip away, and autoimmune disease can kick in. That may be why "the postpartum period, particularly after the first pregnancy, represents a strong risk" for the onset of RA—a fact I didn't know during all my years of disease, and not common knowledge even now. The basketful of probable causes for postpartum onset includes a sudden drop in anti-inflammatory steroids (which Philip Hench tried to boost with his new discovery cortisone). Most likely my inflammatory immune cells waited in the wings during pregnancy, as they were supposed to, then jumped back stronger after birth, turning to joints near at hand.

Apparently it wasn't so much pregnancy as maternity that made me sick—which lends weight to my other old suspicion about RA's cause: that my anxious maternal mind was acting on my body. These days I'm more likely to say my anxious immune cells were acting on my body, but back then, like Dorothy Hodgkin, I came to see myself, with a good deal of blame attached, as "a young woman, under some stress."

This is the final story I have to set straight.

Late one night in 1969, just when John was wrapping up an essay with the words "human trouble," I hollered, "What the hell!"

"Already?" he called back. "But you're not due for weeks. We don't even have the car seat clean."

"Contractions starting. Let's get *going*."

Our VW bug took off with a garage-sale car seat caked in some other baby's leftovers, a passenger unfit for the lap belt, and a driver intoning "Breathe! Breathe!" As we swept past grazing mares on Sand Hill Road, we were clocking contractions three minutes apart, and by the time I got settled in Stanford Hospital, labor pains were hitting me sixty seconds on, sixty off, holding that tempo from afternoon to dark, until the bleaker hours before dawn, into daybreak and full morning sun, heading toward noon. After twenty hours I lost all thought for the baby, except pull it out and leave me alone.

She almost did leave me alone. Born near noon, she went seven minutes without breathing, then coughed into life with just seconds to spare. When the buzz of emergency equipment stopped with her first yelp, I dove into a swift, grave sleep.

Hours later I came out of it in a different room, staring at a figure on the other bed. The shoes were John's. Of all people it was John. A sudden compassion in his eyes didn't make sense at our age: maybe a message from years ahead.

"I love you. How are you?" he said.

"Where's the baby?"

"OK."

"Where?"

"In a special nursery."

"But she breathed."

"That's right. The pediatrician's meeting us later."

"Oh," eyeing a fruit bowl. "They're geniuses here!"

"Well, it's a famous medical center." John smiled.

"The watermelon, I mean," picking a rich, pink slice. "Special nursery?"

"Let's go," John said and set me in a wheelchair. "It's intensive care."

"For breathing problems?"

"For jaundice."

"Is jaundice bad? Doesn't sound bad."

John picked up two surgical masks to enter the special nursery, where the babies, hooked up to tubes, bleated as one, yet the parents knew their own little lambs. A nurse handed us ours. Rocking this marvel softly, I looked upward at John, and that instant he took a snapshot, a picture of alarm. I had just seen the mustard skin of jaundice and heard it might cause chronic damage. Chronic sounded cruel.

Someone came to take a blood test, puncturing the baby's heel. I noticed a half-dozen holes and grabbed the baby's other foot—in that heel too. The holes meant jaundice was serious.

I didn't want to leave her, but a sharp-minded pediatrician motioned us back to my room. Her no-nonsense look was half the reason we'd chosen her. We also wanted a woman doctor, not easy to come by in '69. Now she was standing by the bed, and John stretched an arm across my shoulders so quietly it was plain he'd already talked with her. I was the one getting briefed.

"First of all we have to watch the jaundice," she said. "The bilirubin level is extremely high." No questions popped through my mind. Then one did but stopped short of getting asked: What's "first of all"?

"Then there's the transfusion we're waiting to do." I must have looked blank because she explained. "Bilirubin is a toxin from red blood cells breaking down. If the liver can't get rid of it, a transfusion will. But we try to avoid transfusions," she said quietly. "There's a real mortality risk." John was rubbing my shoulder. I couldn't see his face.

As soon as they left, I watched quiz programs, a Paul Newman movie, ads more local by the hour, until the night nurse asked, "Want to try some sleep?" Not me. Not now.

Early the next morning I was back in the special nursery, where a resident told me he'd done exchange transfusions during the night, twice replacing every ounce of baby blood. "Why'd she need them?" I whispered.

"Because the bilirubin rose to danger level."

"What . . . danger?"

"Brain damage," he said. I managed to ask how they counted the danger level, and he gave me a "plus-or-minus" number. How high was hers? A number far above the plus.

John steered me from the nursery back to my room. During all this time I never held the baby there or nuzzled her head minus a surgical mask.

Where was my travel bag, packed in advance with things I didn't need, like a nice nightgown and a comb? I was after Dr. Spock's *Baby and Child Care*, to look up "brain damage," which I found under "Special Problems," along with "Separated Parents," "The Working Mother," and "The Fatherless Child." Spock said brain damage was "caused, for example, by insufficient oxygen reaching the brain during birth." So the baby had *two* chances for brain damage—from not breathing and from jaundice—and either might lead to "real mental slowness." My humane hero told me that some children grow "brighter, shorter, or taller than average." Likewise a brain-damaged child simply learns "at a slower rate than average."

At midnight the pediatrician shook me awake: a third exchange transfusion. Our baby—not yet named because not yet in our hands—had all her blood replaced with someone else's three times in her first two days. I wondered fiercely how long they'd waited this time. Then I found out the pediatrician had raced to the hospital after midnight, a faraway donor had given late-night blood, an ambulance rushed it down the freeway.

My eyes turned up and stayed glued to local ads.

At home John too had such trouble sleeping he got to the hospital early and came up behind some doctors on daybreak rounds. One of them pointed through the glass at an incubator. "This one had three exchange transfusions in less than thirty-six hours. Not expected to make it." They moved two steps to the left, "This one . . . ," and then on.

John reached the doctor's shoulders and spun him around. "What do you mean, not expected to make it?"

"No one was saying that."

"The baby. On the right."

"We're observing a different one."

The school of doctors skittered past. John hurried to my room. "Mary."

"What?"

Long beat. "Remember they made you take off your ring in the labor room? I can't find it." A wedding ring etched with words from a Mozart song. Exsultate, Jubilate, Latin for untarnished joy. "Exult, Rejoice."

"Maybe in a pocket? Anyway, it doesn't matter now."

"It does. It's gone."

Later in the nursery, with the still-unnamed baby of tubes and heel holes, I too guessed she might not make it, though I hadn't overheard doctors on rounds. For days nothing mattered except each hour looping into another one. Finally, after all the transfusions, she looked a little less yellow. I read Spock again on brain damage, and after a week the three of us went home. We gave her a name.

Once at home I started doing the job of mothering righter than right, minus skill, having taken my entire training on a plastic doll at the American Red Cross. I was so anxious to comfort the baby I just kept nursing through colic all day and night. Nursing with bad posture must have strained my wrists. That's what I thought.

Now I'm reading research on an outcome of nursing that's new to me: "It is the women who breast-feed after their first pregnancy who are at the greatest risk" for RA. An abrupt rise in pro-inflammatory prolactin—a hormone from breastfeeding—is thought to increase RA's chances. Not posture, but prolactin. I'd thought the weak link was mine. Now research wheels everything around.

Back then I fell into a certain lunacy after labor. I kept calling the hospital to ask, "Has anyone found the ring I lost in the labor room?" because I needed its Latin inscription, Exsultate, Jubilate, at home. One night I listened to the words of Mozart's song, starting with "Rise up in gladness." Then I turned to John, barely whispering, " 'Exult, Rejoice' is gone, I think, for good."

By then I'd lost strength and spirit, put on weight and fright, felt emptied out, fumed at John for bouncing back. My briefly scribbled diary shows I hardly slept for months, even when the baby did. Bogged down with fear for her, I neglected to sing in the rain. I didn't know how to help a child I loved who hadn't breathed enough oxygen.

In that diary I wrote a few words dated July '69, a month after the birth: "My sin: I fall to pieces." At some level I eventually began believing my falling apart brought my body's trouble.

But hold on. I can't leave the old belief in place, now that I've seen the burden of blame and shame laid on my disease. Back in 1969 it was acceptable to make RA a mental ailment, to suspect the patient far more than any stress watch should. Physicians did tag RA psychosomatic. Researchers did say female and Jewish patients exaggerate, exacerbate, even earn their illnesses. Back then I was handed every chance to think my own thin-skinned psyche had attracted a disease. Only now, as I fold the whole story into its times, does everything seem less wrongful on my part.

Now I see that the diary goes on ecstatically:

> This child—purrs. She purrs when TV pictures show astro-
> nauts landing on the moon. They've been floating in
> zero gravity, what a release, listening to earth:

Houston: You're looking good here.
Tranquility Base: A very smooth touchdown.

A very smooth touchdown was all I wanted for her. Awhile later I
wrote: "She smiles ear to ear. She pants with excitement, and heaves a
sigh." Then I added, knowing Biafran babies were starving at the time,
"Please let this one grow up safe."

On another page of the little notebook, I find a longer scrawl—oh,
no! I didn't know I actually recorded this moment:

> Late at night I felt a lot of pain in my left wrist and woke
> John. I sat up from 2 to 6 and finally it felt better. At noon
> we went to see an on-call doctor at the Palo Alto Clinic.
> He put a shot of steroids right in the joint. It was terribly
> painful. When we got home the local anesthesia wore
> off, and I was crazy with pain. Took pain pills and finally
> codeine—double doses haven't relieved it. It's got to
> get better soon. I can't stand much more of the pain.

My memory of this is completely different. All I recall is that about a
week after childbirth I came awake suddenly with wrists hammering
and figured my faulty nursing posture had strained them. I supposed
the trouble to be muscle fatigue and the cure a wrist brace. Memory
plainly erased the crazy, unstoppable excess of pain, along with when
it began.

Right away I check some photocopies from my medical record and
notice something I failed to see before, something in a doctor's first
view of my swollen wrists:

> Patient was seen as an emergency last weekend for a
> painful left wrist. No other joint problems, no prior joint
> problems, no real injury to account for her problem. She
> has been busy being a housewife and caring for a small
> child. Impression: Suspicion of early rheumatoid arthritis.
> Date: 10 September '69.

I'm struck also by the first record from my own rheumatologist, and
not just by the "suspicion" I didn't suspect:

> She put up with this pain in her wrist but then it grew
> quite bad. . . . Diagnostic Impression: Probable rheuma-
> toid arthritis.
> Date: 18 September 1969.

Really? Those were the dates? Childbirth in June and rheumatoid arthritis in September? But I've always said—even published the
words—"a week later." So my memory foreshortened the time from
delivery to onset by three months. It fastened the disease right onto the
childbirth.

For years I'd lost sight of the actual onset and never considered
doing medical research. Now to recall my thinking at the time is to
see the magic involved. When my wrists started aching some months
after a touch-and-go birth, after dangerous jaundice and transfusions,
followed by anxious waiting for infant sit-ups and stand-ups, my imag-
ination took to aligning all these events. I arrived at a plea, a prayer
countless parents have resorted to, for relieving a baby from common
ills and unfamiliar dangers. At the time I thought: If I accept RA, no fuss
about pain, then any angel of anatomy ranging through my humdrum
household might pass over the baby's little room. I even thought of the
terms: I'm a first-time mother with human trouble. I'm the one already
hurt, so *leave her be.*

I kept this plea in my bones—it ran that deep: Let her alone. That's
the deal.

As the early months went past, my painful joints felt bargained
for. Then the bargain stopped making sense, and the enigma of onset
stopped mattering. For I grew certain that Dr. Spock and the bilirubin
level had spooked me about the baby's brain. In her next seasons Sarah
proved the danger was done with, and a gladdening gathered around
this new person in our world. The first time she ran toward me crying,
"Mommy! Mommy!" (I can hear it still) and landed wildly in my arms,
I was all one smile.

Only now can I lighten the imprint of an idea that troubled the ear-
liest days and stayed in my mind—an idea that threaded childbearing
into the joints' bitter pain. Someday a discovery might show how close
that connection may be. For now the causes of RA stay intricate and
mostly unknown, but that won't stop anyone from grasping at ratio-

nales. At one time or another I held notions of disease-determining pregnancy, prenatal allergic reactions, psychosomatic dejection, postural faults, and bargains with an Angel of Anatomy. Now, finally, the history I've released has lessened the force of those notions and opened a new beginning.

I settle in my favorite armchair, both of us shiny with wear, and rethink the purpose, if any, of my having RA all these years. At the very least it gives me an insider's chance of exposing its past. At most it allots me a share of human misery, tests my love of living. It shows that curing runs too far ahead to count on—but healing just keeps working away, no matter what, through history.

I slip out of the armchair and step slowly around the room. Reaching the stereo, I'm glad to play again, these many years later, Mozart's *Exsultate, Jubilate*:

> Exult, Rejoice,
> Rise up in gladness
> at the end,
> You who lived
> till now
> in fear.

With the words still in my ear I move to the window and take a good look outside. In the coming dusk the wind sends a willow branch this way and that, like a kite in the hills. I sniff at rain. Hour by hour color will climb through matted brown grass until the ground grows close to green. It's a conversion, if not a cure. For a long time I peer at the willow and the windblown hills, at the rising gladness there.

Retrospect

It's taken a long while to travel all the way around my joints. Now I know my story is what has happened to them.

At the start they got hurt, and I had to get wise. When that wasn't enough, I got help. Then I got back and got past. In the end the surprising discovery came from history.

That it can heal.

It can heal by placing the life you live within a broader timeline. It can prove that you're not alone or at fault. It can bend the arc of your condition, until one day you wake up in the selfsame body but somewhere new. The arrival may come around to the beginning, as mine did, or end up at some other place. Surely any journey makes life livelier and loopier than staying put. So I wouldn't unpack just yet.

Now that I've gone the circle, I can see the story from another side, flipped around. Isn't this finally the new view I've been looking for all along? To know a life as it is, and what it would miss . . . *without* RA?

Without RA I would never say thanks to joints for keeping me on the go. I wouldn't ever look back through them or give memory a reason to take hold. Without memory I would never have seized on a personal voice that started me thinking as a writer.

Without RA I wouldn't find the patience that comes with pain, not to say with life. I wouldn't pity my body for the harm RA did to it, only judge what I did to it. I wouldn't learn to accept losses . . . oh, I never did learn that.

Free of RA I wouldn't watch my friends leaning closer to catch unspoken needs. I wouldn't take lessons from my brother's strengths, or stand in awe of my mother's suppleness, or honor my father's choice to overwater plants because anything can die, he believed, at any hour.

In the absence of illness I wouldn't soak my own begonias to prolong their time.

Without pokey joints I wouldn't have a decent reason for resenting speediness in John. Without needing a hand I wouldn't know the demands placed on him or our ways of pulling together. Without stumbling I'd never earn his lifesaver skill of grabbing my arm, his "Come along with me, Miss." Subtracting stiffness I might not think to admire the resilience he keeps bringing out in me.

Take away ungainly feet, and I'd miss the gracious way Sarah and Scobie support my steps and my dignity. Shake off weak hands, and I'd forego Alek taking the pull of a kite for me, his easy voice asking, "How you doing, Ma?" I'd lose the lighter spells, when he and Sarah snap their fingers twice, meaning present company just made an odd remark. Without a rigid frame I wouldn't stand in awe of fingers that snap twice or feel so goofily grateful they let me into their game.

Without pain at hand I might escape the urge to share in human suffering. Without complaints of my own I might dismiss an Angel of Anatomy.

Without jalopy joints there's no way to guess what I'm made of or how many bang-ups I can withstand. Without these old connectors no way to hold together on the hard way home.

Without the life I live I'd miss one last thing. Whenever pain lets go a little and stiffness releases, the sweet plain world comes nearer, more intense and eager, like stillness touching the ear after cries and shouting.

Notes

The last word or phrase of a quotation appears in italics, followed by the citation. For author information see http://bss.sfsu.edu/felstiner.

Preview

xi *arthritis*: See Kate Lorig and James F. Fries, *The Arthritis Helpbook*, 4th ed. (1995); James F. Fries, *Arthritis: A Take Care of Yourself Health Guide for Understanding Your Arthritis* (1999); Arthritis Foundation, *Primer on the Rheumatic Diseases*, 12th ed. (2001); Gene Hunder, *Mayo Clinic on Arthritis* (1999); Johns Hopkins White Papers, *Arthritis 2005* (2005); Derrick Brewerton, *All about Arthritis: Past, Present, Future* (1992); Thomas F. Lee, *Conquering Rheumatoid Arthritis: The Latest Breakthroughs and Treatments* (2001).

xiv *cover stories*: Jerry Adler, "Unlocking the Mysteries of Arthritis," *Newsweek*, Sept. 3, 2001; Christine Gorman and Alice Park, "The Age of Arthritis," *Time*, Dec. 9, 2002.

Part I: Getting Hurt

1 *"signified by pain"*: Adrienne Rich, "Contradictions," no. 7, from *Your Native Land, Your Life* (1986), in *The Fact of a Doorframe: Selected Poems 1950–2001* (2002), 205.

Shock, 1969

8 *"sedition"*: Thomas Hobbes, *Leviathan* (1651), ed. Richard E. Flathman and David Johnston (1997), 9.

9 *medical chart*: All quotations courtesy of Palo Alto Medical Foundation, Palo Alto CA.

Tops, 1959–69

13 *"brainy"*: "Look What's Going on at Radcliffe!" LIFE, Jan. 4, 1963, 66.

15 *"intellectual life"*: Stephen Jencks, "Coeducation and Monasticism in the Houses," *Harvard Crimson*, May 21, 1963.

16 *"anywhere but sick"*: Flannery O'Connor, quoted in Hilton Als, "This Lonesome Place," *New Yorker*, Jan. 29, 2001, 87.

18 *"her children's care"*: Benjamin Spock, *Baby and Child Care* (1968), 563.

Fatigue, 1971–74

21 *"unknown before in history"*: Kate Millett, *Sexual Politics* (1970; 2000), 363.

Promises, 1975–76

27 *Salomon: Charlotte: A Diary in Pictures by Charlotte Salomon* (1963).

29 *"Male Careers"*: Arlie Hochschild, "Inside the Clockwork of Male Careers," in Florence Howe, ed., *Women and the Power to Change* (1975), 47–80.

29 *gonorrhea*: Boston Women's Health Collective, *Our Bodies, Ourselves* (1976), 174.

Alternatives, 1979

33 *"the presidency"*: Susan Sontag, *Illness as Metaphor* (1978), 84.

33 *twelve thousand people*: Roy Porter, *The Greatest Benefit to Mankind: A Medical History of Humanity* (1998), 687.

34 *"heroic medicine to cure"*: Regina Markell Morantz, "Nineteenth-Century Health Reform and Women," in Guenter B. Risse, Ronald L. Numbers, and Judith Walzer Leavitt, eds., *Medicine without Doctors: Home Health Care in American History* (1977), 89.

34 *"mistreatment"*: "The Mistreatment of Arthritis," *Consumer Reports*, June 1979, 340–43; "The Proper Treatment of Arthritis," *Consumer Reports*, July 1979, 391–93.

35 *"chronic ailers"*: Norman Cousins, *Anatomy of an Illness as Perceived by the Patient* (1979), 45, 87, 95.

35 *"decaying selves"*: Ivan Illich, *Medical Nemesis: The Expropriation of Health* (1976), 134–35, 154.

36 *"depression"*: James F. Fries, *Arthritis: A Comprehensive Guide* (1979), 90.

Part II. Getting Wise

39 *"meant to be gagged"*: Rich, "Contradictions," no. 18, in *Fact of a Doorframe*, 208.

Inflammation, 1980–84

42 *"jaundice . . . to the doctor," "the mother," "30 minutes"*: Benjamin Spock, *Baby and Child Care*, rev. ed. (1976), 5, xix; Spock, *Baby and Child Care* (1968), 143.

43 *turgor*: Aulus Cornelius Celsus (fl. 20–30 AD), *De Medicina*.

44 *painting at the Min*: William Hoare, *Dr. Oliver and Mr. Peirce*, 1742.

44 *"high colleges"*: Paracelsus, quoted in Alan G. R. Smith, *Science and Society in the Sixteenth and Seventeenth Centuries* (1972), 135.

44 *"declining life," "on that account"*: Jane Austen, *Sense and Sensibility* (1811; 1990), chap. 8, p. 32; Jane Austen, *Persuasion* (1818; 1994), chap. 17, p. 101. See also George D. Kersley and John Glyn, *A Concise International History of Rheumatology and Rehabilitation* (1991), 21–29.

Immunity, 1985

48 *immune system*: See Robert S. Desowitz, *The Thorn in Starfish: How the Human Immune System Works* (1987), 53; Emily Martin, *Flexible Bodies: Tracking Immunity in American Culture from the Days of Polio to the Age of AIDS* (1994), 92.

50 *ban Jews*: Dan Oren, *Joining the Club: A History of Jews and Yale* (1985), 41.

Shame, 1986

52 *1986 report:* "Census Study Reports One in Five Adults Suffers from Disability," *New York Times,* Dec. 23, 1986.

52 *"major diseases":* Fries, *Arthritis: A Comprehensive Guide,* 5, 3.

53 *13 percent of Americans:* Andrew M. Pope and Alvin R. Tarlov, eds., *Disability in America: Toward a National Agenda for Prevention* (1991), 57, 188.

53 *1983 National Health Interview Survey: Current Estimates from the National Health Interview Survey, United States, 1983* (1986), 80–87.

53 *"laughable":* Virginia Woolf, "On Being Ill," in *Collected Essays* (1967), 4: 194.

53 *"language is learned," "to have doubt":* Elaine Scarry, *The Body in Pain: The Making and Unmaking of the World* (1985), 4, 13.

54 *"deathbringing speech":* John Felstiner, *Paul Celan: Poet, Survivor, Jew* (1995), 114.

Stiffness, 1987

56 *"tormented be":* Ben Jonson, *On Lord Bacon's Birthday,* lxx.

56 *"out of joint":* William Shakespeare, *Hamlet* 1.5.206.

57 *TB:* Sheila M. Rothman, *Living in the Shadow of Death: Tuberculosis and the Social Experience of Illness in American History* (1994), 184–85.

57 *twenty million:* Brewerton, *All about Arthritis,* 52.

Distrust, 1987–88

63 *"jealousy, despair":* Arthur Kleinman, *The Illness Narratives: Suffering, Healing and the Human Condition* (1988), 45.

64 *divorce, remarry:* Michelle Fine and Adrienne Asch, eds., *Women with Disabilities: Essays in Psychology, Culture, and Politics* (1988), 13, 22.

Morbidity, 1988

68 *menoboomers:* Rose Weitz, ed., *The Politics of Women's Bodies: Sexuality, Appearance, and Behavior* (1998), 242.

69 *constant noise:* Herbert Weiner, *Perturbing the Organism: The Biology of Stressful Experience* (1992), 192.

Mortality, 1989

76 *1989 studies:* See studies in *Scandinavian Journal of Rheumatology* supp. 79 (1989).

Part III. Getting Back

79 *"outwit rheumatoid arthritis":* Henry Roth, *Mercy of a Rude Stream* (1994), 3: 31.

Access, 1993

81 *"battling cancer":* Audre Lorde, "Living with Cancer," in Evelyn C. White, ed., *The Black Women's Health Book* (1990), 34.

81 *"deviant":* Susan Sontag, AIDS *and Its Metaphors* (1989), 25.

82 *quotas to support the disabled:* Christopher R. Jackson, "Infirmative Action: The Law of the Severely Disabled in Germany," *Central European History* 26, no. 4 (1993): 417–56.

83 *"public and us"*: Quoted in Joseph P. Shapiro, *No Pity: People with Disabilities Forging a New Civil Rights Movement* (1993), 22.

84 *Het Dorp*: See Irving Zola, *Missing Pieces: A Chronicle of Living with a Disability* (1982).

Despair, 1993

87 *"mercy to which it leads"*: C. S. Lewis, *The Problem of Pain* (1973), 98.

87 *"diseases do abound"*: Shakespeare, *A Midsummer Night's Dream*, 2.1.105–7.

87 *"joint-racking Rheums"*: John Milton, *Paradise Lost*, book 11, line 488.

87 *"redness and swelling"*: John Sydenham, quoted in W. R. Bett, *The History and Conquest of Common Diseases* (1954), 116.

87 *"one of his shoulders"*: Austen, *Sense and Sensibility*, chap. 8, p. 32.

88 *"out of joint," "taste and see"*: Psalm 22:15; Psalm 34:8.

Moves, 1994–95

90 Salomon: Mary Felstiner, *To Paint Her Life: Charlotte Salomon in the Nazi Era* (1994).

92 Sutcliff: Rosemary Sutcliff, *Blue Remembered Hills* (1983), 86, 88.

92 *voice to arthritis*: See Isabel Hanson, *Outwitting Arthritis: People Talk about Coping with, Controlling, and Conquering Arthritis* (1980).

92 *"should be grand"*: Josephine Miles, "Album," in *Collected Poems, 1930–83* (1983), 209. Copyright 1983 by Josephine Miles. Used with permission of the University of Illinois Press.

92 *"laborious"*: Lester Cappon, ed., *The Adams-Jefferson Letters* (1959), Oct. 12, 1823, 2: 599.

93 *"keep pain / in"*: Jan Glading, "Arthritis," in Joseph L. Baird and Deborah S. Workman, eds., *Toward Solomon's Mountain: The Experience of Disability in Poetry* (1986), 29.

93 *"things as they are"*: Audre Lorde, *A Burst of Light* (1988), 118–19.

93 *"edges that blur"*: Rich, "Contradictions," no. 29, in *Fact of a Doorframe*, 212.

93 *"Articulator of human bones"*: Charles Dickens, *Our Mutual Friend* (1865; 1994), chap. 7, p. 83.

94 *"where I work"*: Peggy Whitman Prenshaw, ed., *More Conversations with Eudora Welty* (1996), 260.

94 *"outwit rheumatoid arthritis"*: Roth, *Mercy of a Rude Stream*, 3: 25–26, 31.

Truths, 1996

100 *"twenty-three million women"*: Arthritis Foundation, "Joint Efforts," newsletter (Summer 1995).

100 CDC *and statistics*: "Prevalence and Impact of Arthritis among Women, United States, 1989–1991," *Morbidity and Mortality Weekly Report* 44, no. 17 (1995): 329–34; "Arthritis Prevalence and Activity Limitations, United States, 1990," *Morbidity and Mortality Weekly Report* 43, no. 24 (1994): 433–38. On arthritis incidence in women see also Johns Hopkins White Papers, *Arthritis 2005*, 1; Brewerton, *All about Arthritis*, 129; Lee, *Conquering*

Rheumatoid Arthritis, 28; Arthritis Foundation, Primer on the Rheumatic Dis-
eases, 12th ed. (1997), 156–57, 246; Charles L. Short, Walter Bauer, and
William E. Reynolds, Rheumatoid Arthritis: A Definition of the Disease and a
Clinical Description . . . (1957), 105, 181; R. G. Lahita, "The Connective Tissue
Diseases and the Overall Influence of Gender," International Journal of Fertility
and Menopausal Studies 41, no. 2 (1996): 156–65; Nortin Hadler and Dennis
Gillings, Arthritis and Society: The Impact of Musculoskeletal Diseases (1985), 6.

101 "capability to reproduce": J. S. Scott and H. A. Bird, eds., Pregnancy, Autoimmunity, and Connective Tissue Disorders (1990), 11.

101 "rates of difficulty": Rima D. Apple, ed., Women, Health, and Medicine in America:
A Historical Handbook (1990), 47, 51.

102 "not been emphasized": "Prevalence and Impact of Arthritis among Women"
334.

102 "apparent for many years": A. J. Silman, "Are There Secular Trends in the
Occurrence and Severity of Rheumatoid Arthritis?" Scandinavian Journal of
Rheumatology supp. 79 (1989): 27.

102 "age and gender findings": J. Paul Leigh and James F. Fries, "Predictors of
Disability in a Longitudinal Sample of Patients with Rheumatoid Arthritis,"
Annals of Rheumatic Diseases 51, no. 5 (1992): 581–87.

102 disabled women: Fine and Asch, Women with Disabilities, 10.

103 African Americans . . . under ten thousand dollars: Pope and Tarlov, Disability in
America, 46–47, 32.

Pieces, 1996–97

107 "female body, out loud": Nancy Mairs, Carnal Acts (1990), 91.

108 "bones, are released": Kenny Fries, Body, Remember: A Memoir (1997), 154.

109 "it's you": Mairs, Carnal Acts, 84.

Wonder, 1941–49

111 "European nations": Jennifer Terry and Jacqueline Urla, eds., Deviant Bodies:
Critical Perspectives on Difference in Science and Popular Culture (1995), 174, 180–81.

112 "Fountain of Youth": Lucas Cranach, Fountain of Youth, 1546, Staatliche Museum, Berlin.

114 "paleopathology": Erwin Ackerknecht, "Paleopathology," in David Landy,
ed., Culture, Disease, and Healing: Studies in Medical Anthropology (1977), 74.

114 "a particular disease?": Joan Brumberg, "Chlorotic Girls, 1870–1920," in
Judith Walzer Leavitt, ed., Women and Health in America: Historical Readings
(1984), 186.

114 "effective cure": Audrey Kelly, Lydia Becker and the Cause (1992), 52.

114 "diabolical trickster": Mary Holder Dietel, The Future Yields to the Brave (1963),
11.

114 "enemy arthritis": Pearson Harris Corbett, Arthritis and I: A Clinical History and
Autobiography (1963), 105.

114 "wishing for the night": Faith Perkins, My Fight with Arthritis (1964), 9.

115 *"soldiering service"*: Ralph Pemberton, "Studies on Arthritis in the Army Based on Four Hundred Cases," *Archives of Internal Medicine* 25 (1920): 382–83.

116 *rheumatic fever*: Peter C. English, *Rheumatic Fever in America and Britain: A Biological, Epidemiological, and Medical History* (1999), 118, 133.

116 *"most disabling,"* *"rheumatic joints"*: Philip S. Hench and Edward W. Boland, "The Management of Chronic Arthritis and Other Rheumatic Diseases among Soldiers of the United States Army," *Annals of Internal Medicine* 24 (1946): 822.

116 *thirty-five thousand disability checks*: Marian Osterweis, Arthur Kleinman, and David Mecanic, eds., *Pain and Disability: Clinical, Behavioral, and Public Policy Perspectives* (1987), 22–25.

116 *German pilots, "downtown for three hours"*: Edward C. Kendall, *Cortisone* (1971), 99, 126. See also G. Hetenyi and J. Karsh, "Cortisone Therapy: A Challenge to Academic Medicine in 1949–1952," *Perspectives in Biology and Medicine* 40, no. 3 (1997): 426–39; Philip S. Hench et al., "Effect of a Hormone of the Adrenal Cortex . . . on Rheumatoid Arthritis," *Proceedings of the Staff Meetings of the Mayo Clinic* 24, no. 8 (1949): 181–97.

117 *"schizophrenia"*: Leonard Engel, "ACTH, Cortisone, and Co.," *Harper's Magazine*, Aug. 1950, 25, 32–33.

117 *"hems of them"*: O'Connor, quoted in Als, "Lonesome Place," 87.

117 *"since for arthritis"*: Mrs. Dick McCoy, quoted in Fred Malone, *Bees Don't Get Arthritis* (1979), 84.

117 *"much worse"*: Dietel, *Future Yields*, 11, 96–97, 185.

118 *victims of these diseases*: Charley J. Smyth, *History of Rheumatology* (1985), 57. See Carl Djerassi, *The Pill, Pygmy Chimps, and Degas' Horse: The Autobiography of Carl Djerassi* (1992); Samuel Rapport and Helen Wright, eds., *Great Adventures in Medicine* (1952), 776.

118 *"little lambs"*: Paul Starr, *The Social Transformation of American Medicine* (1983), 343.

Falsehood, 1950–59

121 *"lived essentially alone"*: Annie Dillard, *An American Childhood* (1987), 194.

124 *"psychosocial factors,"* *"schizophrenia"*: Stanley H. King, "Psychosocial Factors Associated with Rheumatoid Arthritis: An Evaluation of the Literature," *Journal of Chronic Diseases* 2, no. 3 (1955): 289, 288, 296–97.

125 *"cure of rheumatoid arthritis"*: Charles L. Short, "Rheumatoid Arthritis: Historical Aspects," *Journal of Chronic Diseases* 10, no. 1 (1959): 367–87, 380.

125 *"for immunizations"*: Perkins, *My Fight*, 154.

126 *"excessive"*: Estes Kefauver, quoted in *Health Letter*, Mar. 2001.

126 *The Arthritis Hoax*: Public Affairs Committee, ed., *The Arthritis Hoax* (1960).

126 *"our housewives"*: Richard Nixon, quoted in Elaine Tyler May, *Homeward Bound: American Families in the Cold War Era* (1998), 16–17.

127 *"passions of the mind"*: Paul of Aegina (625–90), quoted in Robert S. Hormell,

"Notes on the History of Rheumatism and Gout," *New England Journal of Medicine* 223 (1940): 755.

Pain, 1960–68

129 *"surges of pain"*: Ronald Melzack and Patrick D. Wall, *The Challenge of Pain* (1983), 121. Also see Ronald Melzack, "The Perception of Pain," *Scientific American*, Feb. 1961, 44.

129 *"modern world"*: David Morris, *The Culture of Pain* (1991), 268.

129 *"scientific revolution"*: Melzack and Wall, *The Challenge of Pain*, 233.

129 *"central control"*: Reynolds Price, *A Whole New Life* (1994), 160.

130 *"a communication"*: Thomas Szasz, *Pain and Pleasure: A Study of Bodily Feelings* (1957), 89, 90.

130 *"complained loudly"*: See B. Berthold Wolff and Sarah Langley, "Cultural Factors and the Response to Pain," in Landy, *Culture*, 315–16.

130 *"exaggerated expression of pain"*: Richard A. Sternbach, *Pain: A Psychophysiological Analysis* (1968), 77.

130 *"good American," "neurotic"*: Mark Zborowski, *People in Pain* (1969), 25.

130 *"subjective symptoms," "compared with men"*: David Mechanic, *Medical Sociology* (1978), 188.

130 *"like a man"*: Zborowski, *People in Pain*, 28.

130 *"ethnocultural factors"*: Wolff and Langley, "Cultural Factors," 314.

131 *"self-sacrificing"*: King, "Psychosocial Factors," 288. See R. H. Moos, "Personality Factors Associated with Rheumatoid Arthritis: A Review," *Journal of Chronic Diseases* 17 (1964): 41–55; Richard Totman, *Social Causes of Illness* (1979), 135.

131 *"the genesis"*: J. J. G. Prick and K. J. M. Van de Loo, *The Psychosomatic Approach to Primary Chronic Rheumatoid Arthritis* (1964), 215.

131 *"psychosomatic aspects"*: Short, Bauer, and Reynolds, *Rheumatoid Arthritis*, 170.

131 *"psychosomatic disorder"*: Short, "Rheumatoid Arthritis," 383.

131 *"advance of the disease"*: Perkins, *My Fight*, 142, 9, 16.

Stress, 1997

132 *"calm and peaceful"*: Questionnaire, National Databank for Rheumatic Diseases, Wichita KS (twenty-five thousand participants).

132 HLA-DR: See Bruce Goldfarb, "The Human Genome," *Arthritis Today*, Mar.–Apr. 2001, 54.

132 *genetic influences*: See C. M. Weyand and J. J. Goronzy, "Inherited and Noninherited Risk Factors in Rheumatoid Arthritis," *Current Opinion in Rheumatology* 7, no. 3 (1995): 206–13; Alan J. Silman and Jacqueline E. Pearson, "Epidemiology and Genetics of Rheumatoid Arthritis," *Arthritis Research* 4, supp. 3 (2002): 265–72.

133 *"demented woman"*: Anatole Broyard, *Intoxicated by My Illness* (1992), 21.

133 *"Amazons of Dahomey"*: Audre Lorde, *The Cancer Journals* (1980), 35.

133 *"retrospective necessity"*: Arthur W. Frank, *The Wounded Storyteller: Body, Illness, and Ethics* (1995), 130.

133 *"at the bone"*: Emily Dickinson, "A Narrow Fellow in the Grass," line 24.

133 *"like jewels"*: Song of Songs 7:2.

135 *"exacerbations," "value to the experience"*: Kleinman, *Illness Narratives*, 43, 54.

Part IV. Getting Help

137 *"call it rheumatism"*: Cole Porter, "I Hate Men."

137 *"mile of a joint"*: Philip Hench, quoted in Kersley and Glyn, *Concise International History*, 77.

Family, 1997

143 *"a blustering child"*: Louise Bogan, *Journey around My Room*, ed. Ruth Limmer (1933; 1980), 93.

Partners, 1998

146 *"sexual or otherwise"*: Nancy Finton, "Overcoming Pain with Patience," *Good Housekeeping*, Mar. 1993, 98. Also see Mary Felstiner, "When One of Us Is Ill: Scenes from a Partnership," in Marilyn Yalom and Laura Carstensen, eds., *Inside the American Couple* (2002).

146 *"be a saint"*: Fine and Asch,*Women with Disabilities*, 17.

147 *"are not possible"*: Michael R. Bury, "Arthritis in the Family," in Hadler and Gillings, *Arthritis and Society*, 40, 44.

Time, 1998

149 *"computer chips"*: Anne Eisenberg, "Computers Are Starting to Listen and Understand," *New York Times*, Apr. 23, 1998.

151 *"choose the pace," "time in our society"*: Barbara Hillyer, *Feminism and Disability* (1993), 58, 47.

153 *beginning of ornament*: Robert Hughes, *American Visions: What America's Greatest Art Reveals about Our National Character* (1997), 30.

153 *"mind of its own"*: "Pillow Notes," brochure, July 31, 1998.

156 *twelve thousand people*: "Herbs and Surgery = Danger," *Arthritis Today*, Mar.–Apr. 2000.

157 *"irresistible"*: Margaret Morganroth Gullette, *Declining to Decline: Cultural Combat and the Politics of the Midlife* (1997), 8.

Revolution, 1999

159 *"how arthritis feels"*: Joel Swerdlow, "Making Sense of the Millennium," *National Geographic*, Jan. 1998, 10.

159 *"severest . . . diseases"*: Jerome Groopman, "Superaspirin," *New Yorker*, June 15, 1998, 32.

159 *"twenty billion dollars"*: Andrew Pollack, "Pain under Attack," *New York Times*, June 3, 1998.

159 *hospitalizing twenty-four thousand*: James F. Fries et al., "Non-steroidal Anti-

inflammatory Drug-Associated Gastropathy," *American Journal of Medicine* 91, no. 3 (1991): 213.

160 *billion-dollar molecule*: Groopman, "Superaspirin," 32.

160 "FOR BOOMERS," "PLAY ALL DAY": John Greenwald, "Drug Quest," *Time*, May 4, 1998, 55.

160 *quit work*: Pollack, "Pain."

161 *anti-inflammatory market*, 25 *million samples*, "*pictures of arthritic joints*": Michael Waldholz and Thomas Burton, "Merck and Monsanto to Contest Arthritis Market," *Wall Street Journal*, Jan. 11, 1999; Robert Langreth, "Hoechst to Intensify Marketing Battle," *Wall Street Journal*, Nov. 11, 1998.

161 "*time I've witnessed*": Stephen Abramson, quoted in Michael D. Lemonick, "Arthritis under Arrest," *Time*, Sept. 28, 1998, 75.

162 "*early, aggressive treatment*," *sixteen million more*: Dr. Jack Klippel, quoted in Mary Anne Dunkin, "Where Have All the Doctors gone?" *Arthritis Today*, Sept.–Oct. 2000, 57–59.

162 *thirty-four hundred dollars a year*: *Arthritis Research Newsletter*, July 2001.

163 "*powerhouse in arthritis treatment*": Pollack, "Pain."

163 "*pain wars*": Thomas Burton and Robert Langreth, "Drugs: Two Painkillers Add Up to One Marketing Battle," *Wall Street Journal*, Nov. 10, 1998.

163 "*bruising marketing battles*": Waldholz and Burton, "Merck and Monsanto."

163 "*reinforcements*": Justin Gillis, "New Treatments Ease Arthritis Pain," *Washington Post*, Dec. 28, 1998; Mayo Clinic Women's HealthSource, Nov. 2000, 8.

163 "*targeting every element*": Lemonick, "Arthritis under Arrest," 75.

164 "*ever undergone*", "*seems to have helped*": Joshua M. Smyth et al., "Effects of Writing about Stressful Experiences on Symptom Reduction in Patients with Asthma or Rheumatoid Arthritis," *Journal of the American Medical Association* 281, no. 14 (1999): 1304–9; David Spiegel, "Healing Words," *Journal of the American Medical Association* 281, no. 14 (1999): 1328; Erica Goode, "Can an Essay a Day Keep Asthma or Arthritis at Bay?" *New York Times*, Apr. 14, 1999.

164 "*discourage our stories*": Broyard, *Intoxicated by My Illness*, 52.

164 "*no movie version*": Gullette, *Declining*, 55.

164 "*affirmative ending*": Thomas C. Couser, *Recovering Bodies: Illness, Disability, and Life Writing* (1997), 75.

164 "*illness transitory*": Frank, *Wounded Storyteller*, 115.

164 "*the pretense*": Alison Lurie, *The Last Resort* (1999), 129.

164 "*enable the unfolding*": Shoshana Felman and Dori Laub, *Testimony: Crises of Witnessing in Literature, Psychoanalysis, and History* (1992), xvii.

165 "*when it did?*": Kleinman, *Illness Narratives*, 43.

165 "*oh look!*": Ruth Bendor, "Arthritis and I," *Annals of Internal Medicine* 131, no. 2 (1999): 50–52.

165 *"ruins for my roots"*: Patricia Williams, "On Being the Object of Property," in Katie Conboy, Nadia Medina, and Sarah Stanbury, eds., *Writing on the Body: Female Embodiment and Feminist Theory* (1997), 156.

166 *new consciousness of illness*: See David D. Morris, *Illness and Culture in the Post-modern Age* (1998); Arthur W. Frank, *At the Will of the Body: Reflections on Illness* (1991); Daniel M. Fox, *Power and Illness: The Failure and Future of American Health Policy* (1993), 20.

167 *Huntington's chorea*: Alice Wexler, *Mapping Fate: A Memoir of Family, Risk, and Genetic Research* (1996).

Rights, 1999

169 *Smithsonian conference*: "Disability and the Practice of Public History," May 13–14, 1999.

169 *Linton*: Simi Linton, *Claiming Disability: Knowledge and Identity* (1998).

171 *"without us," four hundred million*: James I. Charlton, *Nothing about Us without Us: Disability Oppression and Empowerment* (1998), 3, 24.

171 BACK OF THE BUS: "The Disability Rights Movement," Smithsonian exhibit, July 2000.

Hands, 1999

174 *"to write," "rheumatism," "the cause"*: See J. N. Tamisier, P. Thomas, and B. Duruy, "Retrospective Diagnosis of Mme. de Sévigné's Rheumatic Condition," and M. F. Kan, L. Beranek, and M. Daudin, "Rheumatic Diseases in Nonmedical French Literature," both in Thierry Appelboom, ed., *Art, History and Antiquity of Rheumatic Diseases* (1987), 78–79, 59.

175 *"change your life"*: Rainer Maria Rilke, "Archaic Torso of Apollo," line 14.

175 *L'Ange d'Anatomie*: Leonor Fini, *L'Ange d'Anatomie* (1949), courtesy of the Fini estate, Paris.

177 *through the skin*: Barbara Ehrlich White, *Renoir, His Life, Art and Letters* (1984), 225.

177 *"poor chickens"*: Y. Saudan, "Did Renoir's Arthritis Have a Repercussion on His Work?" in Appelboom, *Art, History*, 46.

177 *"shortened his brushstrokes"*: Saudan, "Did Renoir's Arthritis," 48. See An-nelies Boonen et al., "How Renoir Coped with Rheumatoid Arthritis," *British Medical Journal* 315 (Dec. 20–27, 1997), 1706.

178 *"groaning to the studio," "nothing but paint"*: Ambroise Vollard, *Renoir: An Intimate Record* (1925; 1990), 74, 72.

179 *"we must embellish," "out of it all"*: Saudan, "Did Renoir's Arthritis," 46, 48.

179 *"world of bridge"*: Alan Truscott, "Humor Isn't Really the Point," *New York Times*, Dec. 16, 1999.

180 *"roam the land"*: Maximilien Gauthier, *Renoir* (1958), 88.

Part V. Getting Past

181 *"new bones again"*: Lucille Clifton, "new bones," in *Good Woman: Poems and a Memoir, 1969–1980* (1987), 118.

Healing

183 "*misinterpreted as hysteria*": Melanie Thernstrom, "Pain, the Disease," *New York Times Magazine*, Dec. 16, 2001.

183 *mortality*: Arthritis Foundation Research Update 2004; S. E. Gabriel et al., "Survival in Rheumatoid Arthritis: A Population-Based Analysis of Trends over Forty Years," *Arthritis and Rheumatism* 48, no. 1 (2003): 54–58; Johns Hopkins White Papers, *Arthritis 2005*.

183 *unaffordable*: Ruth Rosen, "Health Care Dilemma," *San Francisco Chronicle*, Apr. 7, 2002.

183 "*may cause joint pain*": Steve Martin, *Pure Drivel* (1998), 54.

184 *heart attack and stroke*: U.S. Food and Drug Administration, "Public Health Advisory: Non-steroidal Anti-inflammatory Drug Products (NSAIDs)," Dec. 23, 2004.

184 *company research*: Sabin Russell, "Arthritis Drug Vioxx Yanked Off Market," *San Francisco Chronicle*, Oct. 1, 2004; Melody Petersen, "Two Big-Selling Arthritis Drugs Are Questioned," *New York Times*, June 4, 2002.

184 "*ordinary aches*": Burton and Langreth, "Drugs."

184 *Arthritis Cure*: Jason Theodosakis, *The Arthritis Cure: The Medical Miracle . . . That May Even Cure Osteoarthritis* (1997).

185 "*narrative medicine*": Melanie Thernstrom, "The Writing Cure," *New York Times Magazine*, Apr. 18, 2004.

185 *pocketing twenty-five million dollars*: "Ex–Belgian Executive Held in Fraud Case," *New York Times*, May 27, 2001.

185 NIH *budget*: NIAMS communication, Aug. 2004.

185 "*violate the Constitution*": *Alabama v. Garrett*, quoted in Linda Greenhouse, "In Year of Florida Vote," *New York Times*, July 2, 2001.

185 *five million dollars*: Rebecca Trounson, "San Francisco State Settles Disability Suit," *Los Angeles Times*, June 14, 2001.

186 "*attached to a mind*": "Extraordinary Bodies Conference," Arizona State University, Mar. 3, 2000.

186 "*every . . . joint of your body*": Walt Whitman, *Leaves of Grass*, preface (1855; 1985), 717.

187 "*inclined to start writing*": Xavier de Maistre, *Voyage around My Room*, trans. Stephen Sartarelli (1994), 55, 59.

190 "*under some stress*": "Autobiographical Memoirs of Dorothy Hodgkin" (1938), in *The Collected Works of Dorothy Crowfoot Hodgkin*, ed. G. G. Dodson et al. (1994), 3: 809.

190 *women's stories*: On their importance in American culture see Ruth Rosen, *The World Split Open: How the Modern Women's Movement Changed America* (2000).

190 "*more like the picture*": Dorothy Hodgkin, quoted in Sharon Bertsch Mc-Grayne, *Nobel Prize Women in Science: Their Lives, Struggles, and Momentous Discoveries* (2001), 229. Henry Moore, 1978 drawing, courtesy of the Royal Society, London and Henry Moore Foundation, Hertfordshire, England.

192 *On pregnancy, childbirth, and* RA: See J. P. Buyon, J. L. Nelson, and M. D. Lockshin, "The Effects of Pregnancy on Autoimmune Diseases," *Clinical Immunology and Immunopathology* 78, no. 2 (1996): 99–104; N. J. Olsen and W. J. Kovacs, "Hormones, Pregnancy, and Rheumatoid Arthritis," *Journal of Gender Specific Medicine* 5, no. 4 (2002): 28–37; J. L. Nelson and M. Ostensen, "Pregnancy and Rheumatoid Arthritis," *Rheumatic Disease . . . America* 23, no. 1 (1997): 195–212; M. Lansink et al., "The Onset of Rheumatoid Arthritis in Relation to Pregnancy and Childbirth," *Clinical and Experimental Rheumatology* 11, no. 2 (1993): 171–74; J. L. Nelson, "HLA Relationships of Pregnancy, Microchimerism and Autoimmune Disease," *Journal of Reproductive Immunology* 52, nos. 1–2 (2001): 77–84; J. A. P. Da Silva and T. D. Spector, "The Role of Pregnancy in the Course and Aetiology of Rheumatoid Arthritis," *Clinical Rheumatology* 11, no. 2 (1992): 189–94.

192 *"which the impostor?":* Dr. J. Lee Nelson, quoted in Natalie Angier, "Researchers Piecing Together Autoimmune Disease Puzzle," *New York Times,* June 19, 2001.

192 *"transgenerational effects":* Nelson, quoted in Angier, "Researchers Piecing Together."

193 *"normal aging":* Meeting of the American College of Rheumatology, June 19, 1969.

193 *research talk:* Melvin Britton, "Immunologic Differences in Rheumatoid Arthritis," *Annals of the New York Academy of Sciences* 168 (1969): 161–72.

194 *"represents a strong risk":* Alan J. Silman and Jacqueline E. Pearson, "Epidemiology and Genetics of Rheumatoid Arthritis," *Arthritis Research* 4, supp. 3 (2002): 268. See also P. Brennan and A. Silman, "Breast-feeding and the Onset of Rheumatoid Arthritis," *Arthritis and Rheumatism* 37, no. 6 (1994): 808–13.

196 *"mental slowness":* Spock, *Baby and Child Care* (1968), 579–80.

197 *"Exult, Rejoice":* Mozart, *Exsultate, Jubilate,* K. 165.

198 *"breast-feed . . . greatest risk":* Silman and Pearson, "Epidemiology and Genetics," 268.

199 *"smooth touchdown":* "Voice from the Moon," *New York Times,* July 21, 1969.

200 *"a week later":* Mary Felstiner, "Casing My Joints: A Private and Public Story of Arthritis," *Feminist Studies* 26, no. 2 (2000): 284.

Resources

American College of Rheumatology
1800 Century Place, Suite 250
Atlanta GA 30345
800–346-4753
http://www.Rheumatology.org

American Pain Society
4700 West Lake Avenue
Glenview IL 60025
847–375-4715
http://www.ampainsoc.org

Americans with Disabilities Act Office
Civil Rights Division
U.S. Department of Justice
P.O. Box 65808
Washington DC 20035
800–514-0301
Hotline: 800–466-4232
http://www.justice.gov/crt/ada

Arthritis Foundation
P.O. Box 7669
Atlanta GA 30357
800–283-7800, 404–872-7100
http://www.arthritis.org

National Institute of Arthritis and Musculoskeletal and Skin Diseases
National Institutes of Health
1 AMS Circle
Bethesda MD 20892
877–226-4267
http://www.niams.nih.gov

National Women's Health Network
514 Tenth Street NW, Suite #400
Washington DC 20004
202–347-1140
http://www.womenshealthnetwork.org